STROKE PHENOMENOLOGY

WHY A STROKE ON THAT DAY
AND UNDER THESE CIRCUMSTANCES?

STROKE PHENOMENOLOGY

WHY A STROKE ON THAT DAY
AND UNDER THESE CIRCUMSTANCES?

ANNIE ROCHETTE AND PHILIPPE GAULIN

Agio

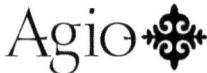

Agio ✛❖✛
PUBLISHING HOUSE
Gabriola, BC, Canada
agiopublishing.com

Disclaimer – *Nothing in this book should be construed as medical advice. You should consult with a qualified medical practitioner about your health concerns.*

978-1-927755-95-2 paperback   978-1-927755-96-9 ebook
Cataloguing information available from Library and Archives Canada.
Stroke Phenomenology is a translation of *Phénoménologie de l'Accident Vasculaire Célébral* (ISBN 978-2-7637-3321-0), published by PUL Presses de l'Université Laval in 2017.

Translation by the authors. Inside page layout by Agio, following Diane Trottier's design for PUL. Cover based on the PUL edition's cover designed by Laurie Patry, with an image montage by Aurel Gaulin.

Agio Publishing House is a socially-responsible enterprise, measuring success on a triple-bottom-line basis. Printed on acid-free paper.   10 9 8 7 6 5 4 3 2 1

TABLE OF CONTENTS

PART 1

INTRODUCTION

This book is intended for everyone who work directly or indirectly with individuals who have had a stroke or who have an interest in this health issue. It is also addressed to any individual interested in understanding more deeply the phenomenological approach. In addition, the content may lead stroke survivors or their families to reflect on their own personal situation from a completely different perspective than that promoted by traditional biomedical discourse. Indeed, the reader might relate his own experience to the case histories presented in the book. This recognition can contribute to reducing the sense of isolation and could help them get through this life-changing experience by encouraging introspection into the stressors associated with psychosocial factors that are present in their daily lives. The circumstances surrounding the onset of stroke have been documented in depth here from a *phenomenological perspective* of many people. These circumstances are presented and discussed mainly in the second half of this book.

From a clinical point of view, the timing of stroke is not trivial. Testimony about the individual events and circumstances of many people provides a better understanding of how psychosocial factors (including the social, affective and symbolic environment) are determinants of the occurrence of this health problem. This advance in knowledge can be considered in order to address these factors during secondary prevention, thus improving existing interventions by promoting a holistic approach to health.

The first half of the book reports on the origin of the questioning "Why that day?" and the second half addresses, from a theoretical point of view, the question of speech[1], phenomenology and medicine as a method

---

1. Note about the translation from the French edition into English: Based on the theoretical framework we are developing, three terms should be clarified to facilitate a better understanding of our translation. We are talking here about the three terms "*parole*", speech; "*discours*", dis-

that would provide benefit with greater clinical use. Throughout this book, the reader will be able to appreciate the importance of the space given to speech, a space that is essential to a clear understanding of the phenomenology of stroke. In conclusion, the two main complementary themes underlying this book, namely the clinical angle (holistic stroke prevention) and the theoretical angle (stroke phenomenology), are used to discuss the essential elements to deepen understanding and that can influence health practises. Finally, an interview guide summarizing the main lines of our phenoanalytical methodology is presented.

ANECDOTE RELATED TO RISK FACTORS

How did we become interested in stroke triggers? Interest emerged during a home visit to meet with a woman in her sixties to assess her condition using a series of tests and questionnaires for a stroke recovery study. This lady was fully involved in the research process and was eager to advance the state of knowledge to finally understand why she had a stroke. Above all, she wanted to know why she had one when she has always adhered to all good and healthy lifestyle habits. She tells me, not without apparent frustration, that all her life she has been careful with her diet, has been active, has never smoked, never drank alcohol. She seemed to have had a life of constraints to make sure she was in good health. Now she is having a stroke. Why me, she said to me? Why not one of those people who abuse life?

These are excellent questions. Stroke risk factors are well documented (Straus, Majumdar & McAlister, 2002) with a history of a previous stroke at the top of the list. Some of these risk factors are modifiable (particularly through the adoption of a healthy lifestyle), such as hypertension, hyperlipidemia or diabetes, while others are not, such as age and having had a previous stroke. The risk of a second stroke in the next two years is

---

course; and "*langage*", language. We will thus say that speech, through discourse, uses language to enter into the life of man. Discourse would be a means which, through the organization of language, expresses speech. It is this speech which, in Heideggerian terms, calls for thought; man taking the floor "*prend la parole*", giving his word "*donnant sa parole*", to respond to this call. In French, the Heideggerian book "*Unterwegs zur Sprache*" is translated as "*Acheminement vers la parole*", while in English it is translated as "Way to the language". In French, the language is more organizational. For his part, Lacan spoke of 'the unconscious structured like a language', and it is precisely in "taking the speech" (*prenant la parole*), in "giving its speech" (*en donnant sa parole*) that man, by way of the psychoanalytic methods, can free self from repressed content. We will have to specify our translation throughout our text.

estimated at 20%, while the cumulative 10-year risk is 43% (Hardie, Hankey, Jamrozik, Broadhurst, & Anderson, 2004).

However, not all people with known risk factors will have a stroke. Some others, with exemplary lifestyle habits, such as the lady in the anecdote above, without any recognized risk factors, *will trigger* one. How is this possible? How can we explain that stroke *triggers* in a person at a specific time in their life, *that day*, when another person is never facing a stroke? According to Saposnik et al. (2006), increased stress is the main trigger for stroke. Indeed, significant stress could trigger a stroke by deficient vasomotor response, heart rate variability or increased thrombolysis (Stalnikowicz & Tsafrir, 2002).

According to the Heart and Stroke Foundation, every ten minutes in Canada, a person suffers a stroke. The extent of stroke incidence in a population over 55 years of age has been estimated at 4.2 to 11.7 per 1000 people per year in a review of 15 population studies since 1990 (Feigin, Lawes, Bennett, & Anderson, 2003). Although this incidence rate has been relatively stable in the past (Barker & Mullooly, 1997), it is expected to increase in the coming years with changing demographics and aging of the population. It is therefore imperative to refine our interventions and strategies for secondary prevention and health promotion related to stroke.

EXPLORATORY PILOT STUDY

From this anecdote emerged a desire to explore the circumstances surrounding the onset of stroke. An exploratory pilot study (Rochette, Gaulin, & Tellier, 2009) on this theme was conducted through a secondary analysis of data collected for a study on adaptation process after stroke. Indeed, participants from a subgroup of the study were interviewed through qualitative interviews that adopted a traditional phenomenological perspective. At the first meeting, which was held at home in the first month after a stroke, participants were asked to tell us about the circumstances surrounding the stroke. Among other things, they were asked to tell us about the month before the stroke, their pace of life, a typical day and whether a particular event had occurred during that time. A brief discussion also focused on the key changes that had resulted from the stroke.

This study did not explicitly focus on the theme of stroke triggers, but on the adaptation process. However, the interview began with an in-depth description of the specific circumstances surrounding the onset of stroke, which allowed the data collected to be analyzed from the perspective of triggers.

Although the specific circumstances were unique and distinct for each of the nine participants in this exploratory study, all spontaneously and freely associated the trigger of their stroke with a conflictual relationship. This association between stroke trigger and conflict-related stress had already been documented in the scientific literature (Engstrom et al., 2004; Koton, Tanne, Bornstein, & Green, 2004). Our pilot study brought new insight on the aspect of secondary benefits following the onset of stroke. Indeed, after the stroke, what was expected in the following days had been compromised or clearly cancelled. For the majority, *what was planned* was overinvested with meaning, emotionally overloaded. The advent of stroke had thus made it possible to temporarily resolve these conflicts, which were tinged with ambivalence.

Upon reading these remarks, a defensive reader could react to these results by arguing that the average person sometimes experiences a conflict situation in their daily lives without suffering a stroke. Absolutely. It would be reductive to state that the conflictual relationship did trigger stroke, just as it would be reductive to say that only hypertension is involved. Like other risk factors, the conflictual relationship may have been present for some time. Thus, it is not a question here of documenting the presence or absence of an objective conflictual relationship in the individual's daily life. What we did was to provide a space for the person who had a stroke to speak out freely about stroke. No questions were asked about the objective presence or absence of conflict. It was the participants who spontaneously and subjectively associated the presence of conflict as a significant component of the circumstances surrounding the occurrence of stroke.

Thus, on the one hand, there was this conflictual relationship charged with ambivalence; a lack of transparency and honesty in the relationship. On the other hand, there were circumstances (e.g., birth, birthday, anniversary, retirement, travel) that contextually exacerbated emotional investment, ambiguity and tension. It was the meeting of all these factors that, together with other genetic or physiological predispositions, favoured the trigger of stroke precisely *on that day*.

QUANTITATIVE STUDY: THE NEGATIVE EXPERIENCE

An important limitation of the pilot study was the small sample size. Obviously, we had the story of only nine people. We therefore thought we would use data collection from a randomized clinical trial with a large sample (Rochette et al., 2013) to re-document the perception of the circumstances surrounding the occurrence of stroke. This study targeted people who had a first mild stroke, returning home within the first month after stroke (note that all contacts were made by phone). They were asked the following question, among several others, at the time of the first data collection: "Is there a specific event (in your personal, family or professional life) that occurred during the weeks surrounding the stroke date?"

Almost half of the respondents (47.5% or 84/177) responded in the negative, emphasizing that no specific events had occurred. However, we found that these negative responses were associated with some interviewers who were not skilled in managing qualitative content. In addition, interviewers who quickly established a relationship of trust, considered respondents' defences and used appropriate strategies by providing relevant space for speech, obtained a positive response to this question. Responses were grouped into categories where the most frequently mentioned themes were the presence of conflict, particularly family conflict, and work-related stress (see Figure 1.1). Some individuals mentioned more than one theme, so the total number of themes was 123 out of 93 positive responses.

We describe this experience as negative because of the large number of responses that invalidate the question by answering: "No, nothing particular happened." In addition, the fact that this response was specifically associated with some interviewers supports the choice of a qualitative method of a phenomenological orientation. We considered then that this method, better adapted and more in-depth, would be able to document stroke triggers. Thus, it would also be possible to allow the person to express himself or herself about potentially contentious content, repressed or protected by defence mechanisms[2] (the issue here was the adequate training of interviewers).

In that regard, particular circumstances emerge from the participant's speech when he/she has the opportunity to express him/herself about them but are rarely addressed at the outset. The individual will tend to look for a cause of stroke among the risk factors recognized and promoted by our society's health promotion campaigns. He/she could also be informed of a cause (based on these risk factors) by medical staff.

However, this does not answer the question: "Why that day?" The stress arising from emotional overinvestment – often repressed, therefore non-transparent – can only be addressed through a structured discourse

---

2.   The types of defences we encountered are outlined in part 2

based on free associations and through a narrative of the circumstances that are specific to that person, but not through closed-ended questioning.

STROKE TRIGGERS: THE MAIN STUDY

This section provides a brief review of the literature on stroke triggers and then follows with the methods used for the main study entitled "Stroke triggers from a phenomenological perspective", the results of which are the pretext for this book. Could the link between stress and stroke on birthday (Saposnik et al., 2006) be related with family conflict, as suggested by the results of our pilot study (Rochette et al., 2009)? Interestingly, the day of birth is one of the non-modifiable risk factors, while the presence of a conflict is a potentially modifiable one.

This main study was conducted with a view to thoroughly document the circumstances surrounding the onset of stroke, as perceived by the individual who had it. It is important to document what is spontaneously associated with the onset of stroke, and how these circumstances may be

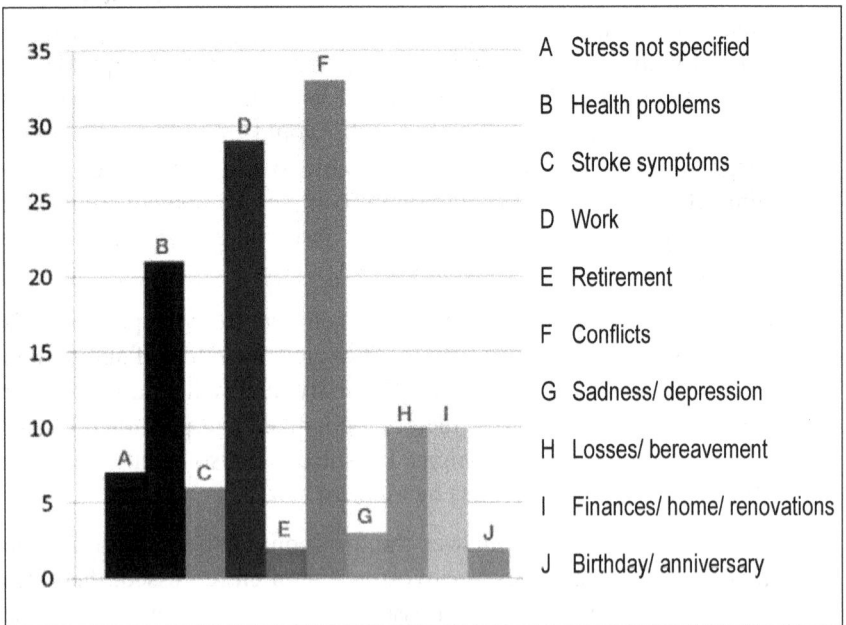

A   Stress not specified
B   Health problems
C   Stroke symptoms
D   Work
E   Retirement
F   Conflicts
G   Sadness/ depression
H   Losses/ bereavement
I   Finances/ home/ renovations
J   Birthday/ anniversary

FIGURE 1.1. FREQUENCY OF THE EVENTS MENTIONED
SURROUNDING THE ONSET OF STROKE

associated with an increased stress as perceived by the individual, in order to take this into account during secondary prevention. Secondary prevention interventions, currently in place in Canada, focus primarily on medical risk factors, treated with medication or support for lifestyle changes (such as smoking cessation, diet or exercise). Psychosocial risk factors (including healthy emotional management), which are perceived as stressors and probably contribute to the trigger of stroke at a specific moment, are not given much attention as they are poorly documented.

Previous work on the theme

This section first focuses on the Human Development Model - Disability Creation Process (HDM-DCP) to properly describe the types of risk factors. Next, available scientific information on potential stroke triggers is presented and, finally, adherence to a phenomenological perspective is justified.

Risk factors according the Human Development Model - Disability Creation Process

The Human Development Model - Disability Creation Process (HDM-DCP) is an anthropological model of human development (Fougeyrollas, 1995) that has greatly inspired the work that led to the International Classification of Functioning, Disability and Health - ICF (WHO, 2001). This model has been used in research with stroke clients (Desrosiers, Noreau, Rochette, Bravo & Boutin, 2002; Rochette, Desrosiers & Noreau, 2001; Vincent et al., 2007). It can be used to conceptualize how stroke, with its various disabilities and impairments, can have a significant impact on the daily life of the individual and their relatives (Rochette, Desrosiers, Bravo, Tribble & Bourget, 2007) - even when stroke is described as "mild" (Rochette, Desrosiers, Bravo, St-Cyr-Tribble & Bourget, 2007). In this model (HDM-DCP), risk factors are described as elements, integrated to the individual, the environment or life habits, that can cause disease or trauma or affect the integrity or development of the individual (see Table 1.1). They are categorized according to whether they are: (1) an organic risk; (2) a risk related to the physical environment; (3) a risk related to social organization; or (4) a risk related to individual or social behaviour. The majority of stroke risk factors fall into the first category (e.g., advanced age, high blood pressure, high cholesterol or obesity) or the fourth category (e.g., smoking, physical inactivity or alcohol abuse). Similarly, as discussed in the next section, the majority of known stroke triggers would be classified under this fourth category and more specifically under conflict risk.

TABLE 1.1

Nomenclature of risk factors according to the four main categories of the Human Development Model - Disability Creation Process

1. ORGANIC	2. PHYSICAL ENVIRONMENT	3. SOCIAL ORGANIZATION	4. INDIVIDUAL AND SOCIAL BEHAVIOUR
Hereditary	Flora and Fauna	Socioeconomic	Traditions
Prenatal	Natural phenomena	Organization of services	Conflicts
Perinatal	Geography	Working conditions	Violence
Infectious	Human accommodations		Nutrition
Health status and physical condition	Sanitation		Use of toxic substances
Development	Technology		Hygiene
			Emotional behaviors
			Behaviors arising from the personality

What we know about triggers

This section presents the few studies that have been identified on stroke triggers. Six studies were identified, including the one that served as a pilot study for the current study.

Haapaniemi et al. (1996) interviewed 723 patients (28.6% female) – or their families – aged 16 to 60 years, within 48 hours of admission for ischemic stroke. The main objective of the study was to determine whether the trigger of stroke differs by day of the week (weekend or leave versus working weekday). Second, the authors also aimed to establish lifestyle habits (data were collected on hypertension, heart disease, diabetes, migraine, hyperlipidemia, alcohol consumption, smoking, transient ischemic attack and oral contraceptive use) that contributed to the trigger of stroke. Multivariate analysis reported that age ranging from 16 to 30 years (odds ratio[OR] 3.13; 95% confidence interval[CI] 1.57 to 6.50), female gender (OR 1.71; 95% CI 1.12 to 2.63) and recent alcohol consumption (OR 2.13;

95% CI of 1.48 to 3.07;) were associated (p value < 0.01) with a greater susceptibility of stroke on weekends or holidays (compared to working weekdays). This study has several strengths, such as large sample size and few exclusion criteria. However, as the authors themselves point out, these results remain difficult to interpret – they suggest an association between alcohol consumption and stroke trigger since Finns generally consume more on weekends or holidays. However, this study does not document whether there were similar circumstances on weekends or holidays, other than alcohol consumption in this sample.

About 10 years later, in a Canadian study analyzing the relationship between stroke emergency room visits (n = 24 315) and birthday, the number of strokes observed was significantly higher (p = 0.009) than expected, reaching up to 30 times the risk of having a stroke on a birthday (Saposnik et al., 2006). The authors discuss the possibility of psychosocial stress potentially present on birthday that would act as a trigger for stroke. They also recognize that birthdays are an unmodifiable factor, but that they are an important contextual element to consider in order to strengthen secondary prevention (such as paying more attention to alcohol or salt consumption or ensuring medication intake), especially on this day for people with risk factors. Since this study used a large database, the variables included in the analysis are limited to those in the database. It would have been interesting and relevant to document the perception of the presence of psychosocial stress surrounding the trigger of stroke in the study population.

In two prospective population-based studies, stroke trigger is associated with family difficulties (Engstrom et al., 2004; Tanne, Goldbourt & Medalie, 2004). The incidence of a first stroke (n = 6 184) was monitored over a 10-year period for a cohort consisting of all residents of the city of Malmo, Sweden, aged 40 to 80 years at baseline (Engstrom et al., 2004). Marital dissolution (divorce or death of spouse) prior to stroke was compared using a case-control sub-sample (n = 3 134 cases of stroke initially married versus n = 9 402 controls initially married). Compared to the married group, the incidence of stroke was significantly higher in the first year after divorce (male OR = 1.23 95% CI from 1.10 to 1.39 and female OR = 1.26 95% CI from 1.12 to 1.41) – after adjusting results for age, country of birth and socioeconomic indicators. Similar results were obtained following the death of the spouse. However, the risk of stroke was not increased in men who had never been married. In the second prospective study of a cohort of 10 053 men 40 years of age and older, where a psychosocial questionnaire was completed at baseline, stroke mortality rates were estimated using the Cox model (Tanne et al., 2004). During the 23-year follow-up, 364 men died of stroke. Among the nine indicators collected, the perception of significant family difficulties (OR 1.34; 95% CI 1.04-1.72), the perception that the spouse and children tend not to listen (OR 1.29; 95% CI 1.00-1.65) and the habit of keeping feelings to themselves during conflict situations with their spouse (OR 1.27; 95% CI 1.03-1.37) were associated with an increased risk of dying from stroke, by controlling for traditional risk factors. These two population-based studies clearly demonstrate a potential link between a family problem and the trigger of stroke. However, we do not know to what extent these family situations have generated stress from the perspective of people who have had a stroke. A positivist approach, where a starting hypothesis has been tested, was used. It would have been interesting to use a constructivist approach where the person who has had a stroke is asked to describe to us, without suggesting answers, the circumstances of stroke occurrence.

In 2004, another study (Koton et al., 2004) used a case cross-over design to identify stroke triggers in a sample of 200 individuals. The main advantage of this design is that the individual serves as a comparison for self by collecting data for different periods of time. Thus, respondents were asked retrospectively from one to four days after stroke, using a validated questionnaire, about their exposure to seven potential triggers in the two hours prior to stroke (case) versus, for the same individual, for the previous day (control). Potential documented triggers were a drastic change in posture following a startle, negative emotions, anger, sudden temperature change, positive emotions, overeating or intense physical exercise. Seventy-six patients (38%) reported exposure to at least one of the seven potential triggers, with nearly 30% for the first three (startle, negative emotions and anger) reported within two hours of their stroke. The combined relative risk was 8.4 times higher (95% CI 4.5 to 18.1) at this moment compared to the control period (previous day). The most frequently reported trigger was "negative emotions". But what were these emotions, anger or startle associated with? Were there any similarities in the circumstances surrounding the manifestation of these negative emotions? Could these stressors have been "prevented" or managed differently? The cross-case study design did not allow to answer these questions.

Justification of a phenomenological orientation

Why favour a phenomenological perspective in this study over a traditional quantitative method using a questionnaire composed of closed-ended questions? This is what this section tries to answer. It is important to remember that participants were not asked about their perception of the possible "triggers" of their stroke, but about the "circumstances" surrounding the occurrence of stroke. These circumstances could give the impression that they are quite trivial and unique to a particular individual. However, the idea here was to document the presence or absence of similarities in these circumstances in several individuals. Thus, the interview mode was anchored in this perspective in order to thoroughly document the meanings (attributive or intentional substance) to which the interviewee relates spontaneously (beyond reasonable conscious discourse) the occurrence of the stroke. The purpose of the interview was to allow the individual to express his/her views on the specific circumstances and socio-affective environment that framed and manifested the stroke. It seemed essential that the interview guide be aware of the defense mechanisms that manage conscious speech to address the heart of demonstrations that were taking place through stroke[3].

The interview based on this theoretical orientation should therefore be able to identify, from the individual's discourse, a network of signifiers[4] (which we will call the vertical axis) that initiate the stroke environment and consequently show what is actually expressed subjectively by the stroke. Thus, the environment of stroke triggers should be identified in the speech of the person who has had the stroke and not based on an interpretation proposed by the interview guide.

In addition, an interview anchored in a phenomenological orientation should highlight a node of meanings (we will call it the horizontal axis) that precedes or accompanies awareness and thematize the *pre-conscious* intentional motives that give meaning to stroke. The important thing here is always to provide an opportunity for the stroke subject to speak out, without suggesting or framing specific content. In this way, it is the essence of the stroke environment that is at stake, that is, what is most important or significant to the network of meanings of the person who has had the stroke.

Summary and relevance of the study

From this literature review, we find that stroke triggers are essential to document as they provide a better understanding of why stroke occurred

---

3.   This will be documented in Part 2.
4.   *Note from translators.* As we will explain in Part 2 in the section on Psychoanalysis and Speech where there is mention of the Lacanian conception.

on *that day rather than on any other day*. This understanding is necessary to identify potentially common stressors in this population on which we could act during secondary and primary prevention interventions so that the person can develop strategies and better manage their emotions to prevent stroke from occurring during these days. We also note that stroke triggers have been studied using a multitude of methods underpinned primarily by a positivist paradigm, which aims to confirm or refute initial hypotheses. The meaning of the day (*that day*) – weekend/leave versus weekday (Haapaniemi et al., 1996) or birthday (Saposnik et al., 2006) - is an interesting indicator to consider. Otherwise, the quality of interpersonal relationships, particularly family relationships – whether it is divorce or conflicting family relationships (Engstrom et al., 2004; Tanne et al., 2004) or the presence of negative emotions or anger (Koton et al., 2004) in the few hours before stroke – has been identified as a potential trigger. Interestingly, a review of the triggers of infarction also supports the few studies reported here (Stalnikowicz & Tsafrir, 2002). In addition, our pilot study was innovative in that all those who had the opportunity to express themselves freely about the circumstances surrounding stroke spontaneously associated it with family conflict; but, more importantly, the trigger of stroke allowed them to temporarily resolve the conflict, rousing thus positive consequences (Rochette et al., 2009).

The idea of using a phenomenological perspective is part of a constructivist paradigm, where we do not aim to confirm or disprove an initial hypothesis, but rather to document exhaustively, and without suggestion, the circumstances surrounding the occurrence of stroke. Family relationships may not be the only associated stressor. Other areas, situations or life events may be associated with stress (understood as an emotional-affective burden) prior to stroke. In cases where the person has had multiple strokes, it is also interesting to document the presence of similarities surrounding these strokes. If there were to be a common scenario of stressors, secondary prevention would be even more desirable to directly target these factors.

Methods: Where does the information reported in subsequent chapters come from?

This section describes the methods used in the main study. The data collected were specifically designed to document the perception of stroke triggers. Data collection was carried out between October 2011 and May 2012. This study was made possible with funding from the Quebec Heart and Stroke Foundation. We also refer to the results of the exploratory pilot study of nine stroke patients (Rochette et al., 2009). Both studies were approved by research ethics boards.

Overall, all individuals with one or more strokes were eligible. To participate, individual had to be able to express themselves in French. Those who had had a stroke secondary to a surgery were excluded for obvious reasons. Also excluded were people over 80 years of age since greater social desirability was associated with older age (Gaulin, Dubé, Hamel & Lefrancois, 2002) and transparency in speech was paramount in the context of this study. Individuals with phasic or cognitive impairments sufficiently important (based on clinical judgment) to prevent them from giving informed consent or actively participating in the interview were also excluded. In the case where the person lived with a relative, the relative was invited to participate in the interview (following the approval of the participant who had the stroke) in order to allow the cross-referencing of the data collected. The relative must also be able to express self in French and give informed consent. We aimed to collect data from at least thirty participants in order to facilitate possible content saturation.

The interview took place at the participant's home between five to eight weeks after discharge from the acute care hospital. All interviews were audio recorded and transcribed verbatim in full.

To facilitate the interviews, we used an interview guide in which the main themes explored were the meaning of the date of the stroke (weekday, weekend, birthday, etc.), relationships with relatives mentioned during the interview (whether or not there is a grey area in the relationship), concerns (what is perceived as a stressor in one's life), consequences (benefits and disadvantages, advantages and impediments) resulting from the occurrence of stroke (what was avoided) and any other issues raised by participants. The interview began with the following short preamble:

As you now know (following reading the consent form), the purpose of this study is to properly document the harmless circumstances surrounding the occurrence of your stroke (or strokes, if any). This interview, which remains confidential and anonymous to the members of the research team, is therefore completely open-ended, that is, it is not intended to identify any cause, reason or responsibility for your stroke, but rather to explore the details, free or indirect associations, surprising or irrational links that are related to the dates, events or coincidences that may be related to your stroke. The purpose of this interview is to try to discover together parallels that can be made about anecdotes outside your stroke, but which, in sometimes surprising ways, can be associated with it. We are not looking for right answers, we have nothing to confirm or measure, we have no analytical grid to fill out, but we just want to chat in an exploratory way to try to make connections that perhaps you didn't spontaneously make. So, we have about an hour or so where I ask you to tell me how your stroke happened and what was happening in your life at that time. Tell me about the day of [stroke date], what was expected in the days or weeks before or after that date, what your stroke prevented, prompted or provoked in a possibly unexpected way. In short, tell me your story...

Data analysis was done as the data were collected, so that content could be validated with subsequent participants (Poupart, 1997). Specifically, the steps in the data analysis consisted of a first global reading of the data recorded on a tape recorder and transcribed verbatim in its entirety. Subsequently, summaries of each interview were written. This step helped to capture the overall meaning of the interview content (Poupart, 1997). At the same time, the verbatim of the interviews was exhaustively coded using a coding grid that was developed as the content was analyzed, thus ensuring openness to new categories related to the themes under study and emerging from the data. Coding and co-coding were done by tagging the content, grouping the categories, and discussing them among team members to arrive at a data classification grid (Patton, 2002). The results of this analysis are presented in Part 3.

In parallel with this data analysis (traditional phenomenological orientation from qualitative methodology), a "phenoanalytical" analysis was undertaken based on the transcript of the interviews. The rationale and methodology for this analysis will be discussed in Part 2, while the results are presented in Part 4, but we can immediately point out that since our first work on stroke, a clinical psychoanalyst has been mandated to review, among other things, the verbatim transcript of the interviews to provide an analysis of the discourses and develop the theoretical framework of the interview guide. Subsequently, the analyst's mandate was quickly defined in terms of coaching and training interviewers. In the main project, the analyst's mandate was specified in two parts, first by inquiring, where applicable, about the defence mechanisms in place and the repressed motions, components or fixations present or repressed in the participants' speech (according to the theoretical corpus of psychoanalysis). Second, the analyst was tasked with developing and undertaking a phenomenological analysis of the content of the interviews, drawing on the work of Edmund Husserl and the clinical work of the Kreuzlingen School, mainly those of Ludwig Binswanger on existential analysis.

PART 2

INTRODUCTION TO PHENOMENOLOGY

SPEECH, PHENOMENOLOGY AND MEDICINE

At the time of the Revolution, many of the first physicians of the modern era practiced by correspondence, without any discussion with the citizen, other than an exchange of personal information. Thus, there is no need to go to the bedside to diagnose accompanied by therapeutics (very simple therapy, which can be summarized in a few rudimentary practices), as this diagnosis can, for a large part of the clientele, be reached without the patient's presence and speech[5].

In a sense, until the end of the 20th century, we could say that medicine generally considered the patient's speech to be unwelcome. The latter was often described as a *poor historian*, i.e., he/she was not in a position, contextually and theoretically, to participate in the process of the diagnosis and the prescription. In short, physicians preferred him/her silent, insofar as his/her word was heard as superfluous, erratic and in search of rationalization extrinsic to medical knowledge and practice. So, silently, he/she became patient, passing his/her tests and briefly answering questions that specifically described his/her symptoms, his/her inheritance and his/her genetic predispositions. The rest of the speech and the rest of the treatment no longer concerned the patient and remained the responsibility of the medical staff.

The rise of the twenty-first century seems to mark a willingness to move towards a novel registry. New visions of practice, called collaborative and partnership visions, attempt to re-establish a system of communication between the patient and the medical staff; this involves giving the

---

5.   See Gaulin, *Le Culte technomédical.*

patient a voice, restoring his/her place in the system and making him/her a first-level partner. New concepts, such as those of patient partner, patient expert or health literacy, clearly indicate this willingness in the medical discourse to partner with the patient, who now enters the care plan as an active element as the one concerned.

But what speech is this about? Do we want him/her to say something, to say what we already know about him/her, to bring him/her back into the position of an object of medical knowledge? Or give him/her the opportunity to express self and be heard from a position as subject, agent of symptom and disease manifestation? But for that to happen, one must be able to hear, that is, to speak the same language. Can the subject be extracted from the patient's position, or is it confined to remaining passive, in the background and being actually patient-passive?

What will we really hear when we give the patient the opportunity to speak? Is the medical staff able to listen to an individual's speech outside the patient's speech, i.e., a speech outside the body being cared for and framed by a care plan? Is the medical staff really interested in hearing anything else from patients?

Many physicians say they are aware of the significant importance of the patient's speech, aware of the importance of the *symbolic* environment (*phenomenological*, which appears and gives meaning) that frames, surrounds and triggers, in the patient's speech, a meaning that is expressed in and through the symptoms and disease. They see this on a daily basis, but remain amazed, not knowing how, methodologically, to support, highlight or use this environment wisely.

At the other end of the spectrum, outside the care plan and the health system, phenomenology, psychoanalysis and existential analysis (which we call *phenoanalytic discourse* for the purposes of the cause) deal mainly with speech. This alternative approach is precisely intended to develop a method that gives the patient the opportunity to speak as an analysand (i.e., as an active part of the treatment) to enable him/her to express directly the essence of the subject as manifested in and through the sense of symptoms and diseases.

Without falling back into the old body/mind opposition, the aim here is to open a dialogue that is intended to complement the two discourses: symptoms and diseases are neither a pure physiogenetic disorganization nor a simple production of the mind; it would be most ridiculous and reductive to reduce them summarily to these expressions. The body and mind suffer in their entirety, in a real body, from a physio, psycho, phylo or phenogenetic heritage, and in the representation that an individual makes of this suffering, expressed by these symptoms and this disease, in an environment, circumstances and a moment that are particular to him/her[6].

The issue is that medicine does not have the time, space and opportunity to listen to the patient's speech; the application of the care plan leaves no other choice. On the other hand, the phenoanalytic discourse is very hermetic, even inaccessible, and can only be located on the margins of the health system, rarely invited to be heard or interested in finding its way around. Are we facing two incompatible realities, two solitudes, or is it possible to open a dialogue about the subject of the speech?

Based on a phenomenology of stroke, an interview guide using speech (working with the practitioner and the partner client) aims to tackle this question and aims to produce a basic tool that bridges the gap between these two approaches, allowing the medical discourse to get to the heart of the matter methodologically, and the phenoanalytic discourse to find a scope of application for its practice.

WHAT IS PHENOMENOLOGY?

Plato launched the idea of a discourse *on what appears* (*phainomenon*), namely what is below the representation that we can have of the world in which we act. Indeed, in *The Republic*, he speaks to us of an *allegory of the cave*, in the sense that man, chained and immobilized in an underground residence, with his back to the exit, would only see the shadow of objects projected on the walls of the cave and would not have access – condemned to a world of representations – to the essential phenomena.

Several centuries later, the French philosopher René Descartes determined this mode of questioning by specifying that any form of affirmation must consider its own experience of the world as a subject. The influence of his "I think", so I influence the order of things, is undeniable. Methodologically (this is a *discourse on the method*), *what appears* must now be considered from the position of the subject who thinks and is included in this world.

In the Enlightenment, German philosophy officially marked the phenomenological approach of its theoretical foundations and engaged in a transcendental discourse, that is, one that concerns the *a priori* conditions

---

6. Environment that we will call *phenopathological.*

of knowledge. In his *Transcendental Aesthetics*, the first part of *The Critique of Pure Reason*, which was originally intended to be called *Phenomenology*, Emmanuel Kant (the 18th century German philosopher) aims to study the *a priori* forms of sensitivity and gives rise to the phenomenological discourse as such. Kant thus lays down the circular requirements of an argument that determines the formal conditions of the experiment while giving proof of its argumentation by the experiment itself. At the end of this *Critique*, in his *Transcendental Theory of the Method*, Kant gives us here to think by distinguishing a rational knowledge by *concepts*, philosophy, in comparison to a rational knowledge by *construction* of concepts. This conceptual knowledge includes its own participation in the experience and refers to the conditions of possibility of this experience. While this Kantian distinction deals with pure knowledge, which is not empirical, we can use it to develop a new distinction that will help us understand a revised conception of stroke.

As well, a few decades later, the German philosopher G.W.F. Hegel proposed in one of his main works, *The Phenomenology of Spirit*, the science[7] of the experience of consciousness and set the tone for the German idealism that would mark the history of the phenomenological approach. In Hegel's work we find this form of "transcendental circularity", and well beyond, at the moment when he poses[8] the thought being in the movement of the thought of the being, thus conceiving *the* system that aims at the unity of the being and the thought in the content of the Thing itself – an element of a transparency in which the thought is deployed in its true sense.

What we must remember from now on is that phenomenology implies the individual's own participation within his/her discourse: something is positioned, posed, attributed in the discourse without the person's consciousness being formally aware of it. We must methodologically focus our attention on the *intentionality* of the discourse, which pushes the discourse to express meaning, to give meaning through what appears in connection with something. Apart from this attention, we can only determine the experience in its beyond, in its representation, that is, outside the experience itself, by *constructing* links from our reason, and we will always be condemned to be right, in the sense of a vicious circle attributed by a reasoning reason.

The thought of Martin Heidegger (a German philosopher who died in

---

7. *Wissenschaft*, not to hear "science" from a scientific point of view.
8. As one of his commentators and translators to French, Bernard Bourgeois would know how to write so well.

1976) has definitively marked the history of phenomenology. In his texts and essays on *Discourse on "thinking"*, *The Thing*, *Moîra* (Parmenides) or *On the Way to Language*, Heidegger indicates the attitude to adopt in front of *what appears* (*phainomenon*), what manifests itself through what gives meaning. He tells us to have the stamina to take under his care what is exposed in the language, and to stick to an in-between. Our discourse must support its position as a fold that accepts what is expressed *by taking in guard* (*noein*) *what is extended in front* (*legein*)[9]. Only in this way can man occupy his mind towards what is worth thinking about. Man must give his speech and memory to thought, be grateful and remember the gift of being called to think[10].

According to Heidegger, this call to thought precedes the Socratic period (Plato) and concerns a guided, influenced conception, motivated by his perception of Parmenides. In this sense, Plato would have already said too much, the world of the idea being an idea of determining representation that does not address the Being or the Speech. The call to thought is indeed launched as soon as man is addressed the Speech, it is a question of folding up into this Speech and not of coming to demonstrate what it means.

Everything that is said outside, below, beyond this folding, this "inter-view", is of the order of representation, suggestion, demonstration, prescription or interpretation and can only be right because it is no longer a question of speech, but of a monologue to know who is right. Usually, the individual who talks to self is always right (he/she can even convince self to take his/her own life). According to Heidegger, man's scientific destiny has turned away and forgotten the fundamental question of his History, that of the Being of the Language, and has thus fallen into the history of a representation of the being. In this sense, *science does not think* and would be unable to do so, obsessed with its technology.

PSYCHOANALYSIS AND SPEECH

But, despite what Heidegger thinks, Freudian psychoanalysis is in an excellent position to meet these methodological requirements and produce a space for *what is extended in front*, on a couch, what is expressed about

---

9. That we will find in Husserl's noetic-noematic structure.
10. We find here all the relevance and rigour of the Hedegerian discourse which shows the common etymological origin, in German language, between thought (*Denken*), gift, recognition and memory (*Dank, Gedanc* and *Gedächtnis*).

speech – although not the same speech here, but two distinct speeches – aimed at distinct project, syntonization and tone. The methodological challenge of psychoanalysis consists in showing (*Deuten*[11]) what is said about the one who gives his/her speech, and to inhabit this space, to stick to this interview, resisting any form of interpretation that would push us to want to understand, know or appropriate any sense of discourse outside the speech and the space of analysis.

But, although we are in an excellent position to hear the subject's speech, the space and time required for psychoanalysis can hardly help us to fulfill our task if we consider the setting of an interview about stroke. For its part, psychoanalysis, neither that of Freud nor that of Jacques Lacan (a French school that began in the mid-twentieth century, which we will use to perfect our method), will probably not be able to help us if we are interested in a phenomenology of stroke. On the other hand, it is interesting to read Freud writings in 1930 that "in a hundred years' time, when the effect of the mind on the body will be better known, some scientist will surely be able to specify that there is a link between a psychological conflict and a brain hemorrhage[12]". So we're almost there.

If we are interested in building an interview guide that leads us to an analysis of the circumstances surrounding the onset of stroke, the contribution of psychoanalysis is undeniable. But, from the outset, our *phenoanalytical* conception places us in front of a dilemma (far from being insurmountable). On the one hand, as we mention, the framework of the interview does not allow us to engage in the space and time required by psychoanalysis, one of the only ways to thwart the defense mechanisms and the resistance of consciousness to the content it tries to repress in the expression of its symptoms. However, we can use the *topology of the unconscious* proposed by the work of psychoanalysis to anchor our theoretical foundations and anchor our phenomenology of stroke[13].

On the other hand, the qualitative methodology of phenomenological orientation analyses (which too often forgets or ignores the philosophi-

---

11. Which is also, or strangely enough, the same methodological issue as Heidegger's.
12. *Le président Wilson*, page 191 (free translation from French).
13. Let us not forget that Freudian psychoanalysis and Husserlian phenomenology (which we will see later) are very contemporary, Freud and Husserl coming from the same province of Moravia, having lived at the same time and having both, precisely at the same time, studied in Vienna, with Brentano, the main Thesis concerning intentionality. Despite their three-year age difference, their life of more than 80 years, Freud never talked about Husserl and Husserl never talked about Freud. If no one is a prophet in his country, it is difficult for two prophets to exist and survive in the same life.

cal foundations of its approach) pays little attention to the *pre-conscious* framework of the interview, i.e., the same defence mechanisms intrinsic to consciousness that make it difficult for the individual to engage in the recognition of the content of his/her speech – as if the person was defending self against his/her own speech. We assume that there is only one experience in the world, that we cannot say anything about it and that we really cannot get away from it. On the other hand, we can talk about it negatively, by denying it, refuting it, trivializing it, ironing it, raving it, making humour without however detaching ourselves or getting away with it, we are then faced with the defense mechanisms of consciousness. We have no choice and we must deal with these defence mechanisms without offending them.

This is why we must revise the framework of the interview, instructed in the work of psychoanalysis on the defense mechanisms of the psychic apparatus, so as not to clash with these defenses, not to amplify its effects by repressing the speech of the Ego, and to hear clearly what is happening to the discourse and the meaningful environment that is expressed through the stroke.

These works of psychoanalysis, this topology of the unconscious, we will not read it strictly from Freud, but rather we will benefit from the *semantic* proofreading and translation that Lacan proposes, imbued with a phenomenological influence (think among others of the collaborations of Maurice Merleau-Ponty and Jean Hyppolite at the Lacan *Seminars*[14]). This translation can only benefit, anchor, moor and refocus our arguments.

According to the Lacanian conception, *what appears* is organized around a network of signifiers that constitutes the Unconscious as a language. A signifier, as such, means nothing; it enters into a *relationship of meaning* in relation to other signifiers, in a chain of signifiers that is language. This chain of signifiers forms a symbolic order from which the individual weaves a web that permeates his/her imaginary order to recognize self and claim a position of subject (which will become the Ego).

In this symbolic order, a signifier, such as first name, gender, date and place of birth, is not trivial. Other signifiers, such as those concerning the date, age, reasons or causes of a parent's death, or those that are recurrent in the speech of those around, as well as those that identify his/her relatives, family, spouse, children and their environment, are just as decisive. All these signifiers constitute the network of meanings that establish the

---

14.   Let us note that Lacan was Heidegger's friend.

background of the subjective (or even imaginary) universe of the subject (consequently of a stroke subject). It is from this network of meaning that the person builds self as an Ego, recognizes self in his/her relationship with others and lives in a world of meanings.

The challenge of the interview is to identify (*showing* would be a more appropriate term in a Freudian dynamic), from the speech that is given, the signifiers according to which the individual positions self, expresses self and constitutes self in a significant environment. The signifiers here serve as symbolic landmarks for living in this environment and describing its field of existence, that is, what it subjectively expresses itself through stroke.

After removing the *subject of stroke* from its usual discourse, which presupposes the phenomenon as an *accident*[15] (which we will call *Gegenstand*) that occurs outside a relationship of meaning, the interview aims to highlight the main signifiers (master signifiers), in and from the individual's speech, that elaborate the meaningful environment that gives meaning to stroke in a particular emotional context, in a particular place and space, at a particular time and date. After identifying these signifiers and the existential dynamics of the main issues at stake here, the interview can then move on to an interview that focuses on the *lively heart of the matter*[16], i.e., the very circumstances surrounding the occurrence of this stroke.

It is imperative that the interviewer be able not to offend or confront the defence mechanisms of the Ego (mechanisms that push this Ego out of the relationship of meaning that is expressed through stroke). It is equally imperative not to clash, insist on or directly identify repressed signifiers who preserve the circumstances surrounding the occurrence of stroke outside the realm of consciousness (let us not forget, and remember, that we are not within a space of analysis that aims precisely to remove these defences and repressions, and that we cannot afford to touch, in an interview, the individual's resistance here). To do this, the interviewer[17] must be on the lookout for the main verbal reflexes that present these defence mechanisms and know how to support them, comfort them, without opposing them. It is necessary to know how to identify these mechanisms quickly and to support them in order not to raise new resistance. The challenge is

---

15. *Note from translators.* In French, stroke is commonly called a cerebrovascular accident for *accident vasculaire cerebral – AVC.*

16. Lively, living dynamic that makes the master signifiers inscribe themselves by associations (displacements and condensations), in a network of decisive significance for the subject.

17.. That is why we emphasize the importance of interviewer training.

to follow the discourse and approve the logic that obviously gets bogged down in negation, denegation, denial, trivialisation, refusal, irony, etc.

Finally, it should be noted that, just at the border between psychoanalysis and phenomenology, just at the borders of the thesis and works of Freud, Husserl and Heidegger, are the clinical works of the Kreuzlingen School, mainly those of Ludwig Binswanger on existential analysis. Educated by the dynamic character that motivates the therapeutics practiced by the clinical approach of this psychiatric school (which benefits from Freudian theory), we can only facilitate and theoretically anchor the development and construction of our interview guide and its methodology.

HUSSERLIAN PHENOMENOLOGY AND SPEECH

But how precisely can we understand, methodologically, the subject of stroke? How can we hear what is expressed in and through stroke? Edmund Husserl, a contemporary philosopher of Freud who has devoted his work to phenomenology, could certainly help us to move forward in our analysis.

According to his thesis, mainly those of the *Guiding Ideas for a Phenomenology*, those of the *Cartesian Meditations* (*Introduction to Phenomenology*, where we find Descartes) and especially those of the *Logical Research*, Husserl bases the phenomenological approach on the notion of *reduction* (which we can understand as a folding). Starting from the principle that we must put in brackets (*épochè*) all forms of judgments or beliefs that the object of the discourse (in this case stroke) is extra-mental (*Gegenstand*) – i.e., existing outside a meaningful, even intentional link – a phenomenological reduction must raise the initial expression of the object as an intentional object (*Objekt*) and take the discourse in the sense of its intentional content. Once this reduction made, we are thus faced with a noetic-noematic structure[18] that brings us back to an intentional act rather than moving away from the demonstration of the real existence of the meanings of the object.

Through phenomenological reduction, the object supposed to be extramental manifests itself as an intentional object (*Objekt*), it subscribes in a meaningful link for consciousness, it raises its intentional content. It is then that a second reduction, the *eidetic* reduction, is able to animate this content to highlight the intentional act as a pure expression of *meaning*.

---

18.   From *noesis* as an act turned towards the object, and *noema*, as an intentional object.

If we are interested in building an interview framework that leads us to analyze the circumstances surrounding the onset of stroke, the contribution of Husserlian phenomenology is fundamental. Thus, if we apply the methodological principles of Husserlian reduction to the phenomenology of stroke, we said that we must first put in brackets (the Husserlian *épochè*, suspending judgment) the tendency to view stroke strictly as a biological, objective, real, simply accidental phenomenon, predisposed only by genetic heredity, outside a meaningful universe or intentional structure. This attitude of restricting the meaning of stroke is, according to Husserlian terminology, of the order of a *Gegenstand*, an extra-mental object that would stand there, in itself, as external to any form of incursion that could eventually lead us to a universe of meanings[19] (*Bedeutungslehre*).

In a sense that bifurcates the judgment that predisposes stroke as an accident with no meaningful impact, i.e., away from terms prejudging stroke such as *Gegenstand*, the interview must be able to give voice to this stroke in order to express the intentional content that is manifested by the stroke. We then make a phenomenological reduction by moving the *Gengenstand* in the direction of an *Objekt*, object of intentional content, which is affirmed in and by the subject's speech.

As part of this orientation, the core of the interview is conducted as an interview that gives speech's space to this intentional content of stroke in the sense of an intentional act (*Inhalt*). We then speak of the discursive effects of a second reduction, an eidetic reduction (*eidos*, essence), which is able to express most of the intentional dynamics that occur through stroke.

THE CHALLENGE OF A STROKE PHENOANALYSIS

If we really want to get into the subject of stroke, it will be a question of showing the language of the unconscious of this stroke, that is, of going in the direction of what manifests stroke (it is not necessary for the subject to be conscious in itself, it is not essential for him/her to know what is present through his/her stroke). The discourse that deals with showing what we are talking about here is called *an analytical discourse*. Although distinct from the formal framework of philosophical discourse, phenoanalytic discourse has its theoretical origin in the transcendental form of

---

19.   In the stroke trigger study sample, very few participants hid behind this tendency to deny by saying that, subjectively, they were not related to the stroke; these participants were the most defensive respondents.

Kantian discourse, namely in its desire to establish the conditions for the possibility of experience. On this subject, as mentioned above, Kant wrote that a fundamental distinction must be made between a rational knowledge *by concept* – the transcendental and phenomenological philosophical discourse – and a rational knowledge *by concept construction* – the scientific discourse applied to a mathematical principle. To be consistent with the goal we have set for ourselves, we must clarify the Kantian distinction by adding a knowledge that is no longer merely rational, but which is the place of exhibition that leaves the concept extended [there ahead[20]] and that takes care of taking it under its guard by giving it a space – the phenoanalytic discourse. It is a question here of distinguishing between whether we are talking about *the exact thing*, or about a system of representation that frames it, determines it and prescribes a meaning for it outside the scope of its experience. All is needed is the stamina to maintain self in the very sense of stroke and stick to it. It should be noted that the phenoanalytic discourse deals with only one thing, what the individual who has had a stroke says about it. It is imperative to stick to this interview, not to say anything more than what is emerging between what is said and what gives meaning to stroke. Apart from that, we find ourselves constructing reasons that will prescribe the meaning of stroke; that is, seeking the meaning of its causes, which, in the end, can only prove us right.

But what do we mean when we talk about the exact thing? To illustrate this, let us take the analogy of medical discourse in the face of the pathophysiological manifestations (symptoms) of stroke. When health professionals receive an individual in the emergency room and see obvious signs such as facial paralysis (collapsed face), inability to lift the arm, vision problems, slurred speech, misunderstanding simple instructions, loss of balance or sensation, painful headaches, etc., they do not take the time to ask self if this individual is aware of his/her condition, aware of what is happening, and give him/her an order of priority that leads immediately to neurology or the surgery. For this to happen, it is especially not essential that public opinion or someone who is not sensitive to the signs of stroke agree or understand what exactly is happening. When these signs are present, two neurologists do not have to consult each other to confirm a diagnosis; according to them, things speak for themselves and are clearly obvious.

The same applies to psychological symptoms, repressed components or predisposing fixations that disrupt the somatic balance or mind of the

---

20. Inspired by both the psychoanalytical couch and Heidegger's *noein/legein* relation.

human being. We know, for example, since Freud's work on dreams, that the content of dreams only makes sense in the dreamer's mind, but the one who is interested or sensitive or attentive to the logical organizational structure of dreams – who conceives the symbolic grammar of dreams that is expressed through displacement or condensations (metonymies or metaphors, would say Lacan) – can hear the meaning expressed by the dream and analyze its content (as with the discussion between our two neurologists, two psychoanalysts do not have to consult each other to agree on this expressed content, *It speaks in the meaning*, Lacan would say).

Thus, it may seem trivial to someone who has not been exposed to phenoanalytical work (phenomenological, psychoanalytical or existential analysis) to find that a man had his stroke on the day of his mother's second marriage, after this individual had succeeded, after many insistent negotiations, in convincing his mother to divorce her husband (biological father of this individual), the day when this other man had to have his front teeth extracted (the same teeth he had, at the age of twelve, accidentally broken to his father while playing a team sport) or the day that this young single woman had her stroke at almost the same time that her younger sister gave birth to the first daughter of her generation or, finally, to note that this individual was showing the first symptoms of stroke when his younger brother signed, in front of the notary, the documents making him the new CEO of the family business.

All of these case histories are classic stroke triggers, processes which we will find in the stories of the participants in our work. The scope and symbolic content of these phenomena may be obvious to those who are able or accustomed to hearing such statements and may seem crazy or surreal to a neophyte.

But what do we hear when we don't talk about the exact thing? Everything is possible here. Outside the exact thing, one can rave, hallucinate, use a mystical link, talk to aliens, predict the future, believe in God, mutilate oneself or commit suicide. It is also possible, as Kant wrote, to construct concepts. What does that mean?

We are talking reasonably here. Our two neurologists speak reasonably, but are [almost] not concerned with the speech of the stroke subject. This speech is of [almost] no use to them to facilitate, improve, refine or develop their treatment plan (which, it should be noted, is most effective).

Thus, this discourse, scientific, proves to be a rational knowledge by constructing concepts using the phenomenon of stroke to make it correspond with something of the order of reality. Science indirectly defines reality and makes the stroke experience coincide, through hypotheses and demonstrations, with its real content (it is at this point that the media often jump at the opportunity to insert the notion of "cause" between stroke and the real content demonstrated by scientific research to draw early conclusions – which is no longer scientific).

By discussing the real relationships of stroke, the scientific discourse can only be right, it has reason on its side. Stroke is indeed a real phenomenon; it is probably one of the most painful and stressful experiences of the existence of reality.

According to scientific requirements, if this concept construction respects its methodology and the rules of reason, i.e., if it is theoretically anchored, objective, rigorous, credible, reliable, valid, meaningful, coherent, innovative, etc., it will consequently be able to identify the real substances of stroke. But we still don't talk about the subject of stroke, and especially not about its cause (which probably only interests the sensationalist press and its readership).

PHENOANALYTIC INTERVIEW GUIDE ABOUT STROKE CIRCUMSTANCES

Subject – It should be noted immediately that our investigation is not limited solely to the field of stroke, that any form or group of conditions could have attracted our attention[21] (our future work will focus on the circumstances surrounding subarachnoid hemorrhage, with or without aneurysm). The reason we have favoured the world of stroke (cerebrovascular *accident*) from the outset is especially because it occurs under the conditions of an *accident* (i.e., by definition, *not essential to the being*), which is fertile ground for an interview surrounding the circumstances of its occurrence, naturally external to intentional content and capable of not confronting the individual's defense mechanisms from the outset.

Let us take advantage of this clarification to open a parenthesis and highlight the influence that an individual's surroundings or symbolic environment can have on his/her conceptions, judgments and beliefs (*Gegen-*

---

21. If, as Freud wrote in 1930, it may have taken 100 years for the scientific community to be ready to consider the influence of a psychological conflict [an intentional structure] that is expressed through stroke, perhaps in another hundred years we can consider the possibility of writing a cancer phenomenology – the ultimate bastion of the sacred in our North American, even Western, technological society.

stände) making stroke an extra-mental phenomenon, genetically predeter-
mined, without external influence on this predisposition. By keeping away
from this *Gegenstand*, we will talk here about *phenogenesis*, i.e., the role
that the environment plays and its influence on the individual's conceptions. The morbid seems to have a decisive influence on the authenticity
of the family inheritance; the causes of death of the ancestors becoming
proof of the purity of the descendants who will die for the same reasons
(although this descendance is from the in-laws or may have sometimes
been adopted). How many times have we heard this kind of discussion, at
the funeral of a family member, saying about the deceased: "He was a real
Jones, he died with his heart"? For many individuals in need of existence,
belonging to the clan becomes something imperative, any reason is good
to identify with it. The major diseases and the purity of the genetic tradi-
tion that is conveyed about them offer a final opportunity to be recognized
and elevated to the rank of full member of this clan (despite the dire consequences associated with them).

As one study participant who had a stroke during a workout at the
gym (and expressed an idea indirectly conveyed by other participants)
made clear: "[...] despite my healthy lifestyle, there was nothing I could
do about it, stroke is genetically programmed, living is waiting for it to
break out. I knew I had had a stroke, I saw my father have one, under the
same conditions."

Guide – To get to the subject of stroke, we can say, briefly repeating
what we said above, that an interview guide must *show us the way* (guide
in the sense of the old French *guier*) to get us precisely to the heart of the
matter. In Heideggerian terms, it is a question of having the stamina to fold
to the subject's speech, that is, to have a true *On the way to the language*.
It is therefore a question of taking charge of *what is exposed*, of giving it a
residence so that it expresses the meaning of its words, a place, a space of
expression that brings it back to its words, that is, to the experience itself
of the words [Kant], without wishing to make what is exposed coincide
with a pre-established theoretical content [a construction of concepts] that
the interview would like to re-find, to justify.

It is therefore a question of *taking charge* by giving expression to
what is attributed by consciousness [Hegel], without it actually being
aware of it. It is in fact a question of the interview guide being able to
give a place for consciousness to express itself, and of the content of the
interview being used to *show* [Freud and Heidegger's *Deuten*] what consciousness expresses to its defending body to enter into a dialogue with the
meaning of stroke in question, to enter into the subject in question [Lacan]

and to interact to avoid the subject being inhibited by the defense mechanisms that the Ego has built itself.

Interview – It should be noted that, according to the methodology presented in the analytical discourse of psychoanalysis and Husserlian phenomenology, the first goal of the phenoanalytic interview is twofold; let us say that it is vertical and horizontal. First, the interview must identify, indicate, show the master signifiers (intentional objects) that vertically trigger stroke at the particular time it occurs, currently in an individual's life; then, it must support, inquire, investigate, from the subject's speech and discourse, the network of meanings (intentional content) that predisposes, organizes, arranges, horizontally, from the experiences lived by the individual during his/her existence, the morbid consequences that the encounter of these current signifiers (intentional objects) has.

When an affective, conflictual and repressed predisposition during an individual's life (horizontal predisposition) encounters a current pre-significant situation (master signifier or vertical intentional object) and the symbolic environment of this individual is inhabited by a phenogenesis insisting on the biogenetic heritage of a specific pathological environment belonging to him/her, we are then in the presence of a trigger of stroke[22].

From the beginning of the interview, a study participant knowingly speaks, as a strange coincidence, of September 23rd, the date of his stroke, as the same date as the stroke that killed his father in 1983. Further investigation during the interview will make him say and realize that at the time of his stroke, in 2011, he was exactly 43 years old, the age at which his father died as a result of his stroke (here, the coincidence was less funny). Vertically, father and son had a stroke on September 23, horizontally, in the subject's subjective existence, the father died at 43 years of age on September 23, an age he had at the time of his own stroke in 2011 (which

---

22. It should be noted that the substrate of the stroke experience is and remains the subject's body in its reality (and in its biogenetic heritage). The meeting of the vertical and horizontal axes is based on the real body of an individual. Stroke is a real phenomenon; it is a manifestation in reality, the body of the individual suffers from it in its entirety, in his/her daily life, in his/her physical and psychological reality, as well as in his/her relationship with others. What we bring to the debate is the fact that, even if stroke is real, it does not change the determining importance of other predispositions that are of a completely different order, symbolic or environmental (as we said, psycho, phylo or phenogenetic). Whether a stroke is a real phenomenon does not make the reality the reason for the stroke, its cause or trigger; as a phenomenon, it cannot be its own trigger, it is influenced by various circumstances outside itself. A phenomenon cannot be its own cause or reason without admitting, a priori, the existence of a principle that is essentially extrinsic to it.

he knew, but unfortunately had forgotten).We will have to come back to the defense mechanisms specific to this interview (most interesting) as well as the intensity of the emotional conflict that linked this individual to his father.

Circumstances[23] – Our pilot and preparatory studies immediately tipped us off to the kind of comments we could hear during our research projects. When asked negatively[24] by the interviewer about a possible meaning that the date of his stroke could represent: "Nothing special happened on March 22nd", a participant in the pilot study explains and spontaneously answers: "No, no, I know that nothing special happened on March 22nd, I remember very well, because that was the date my son killed himself." Invited to elaborate on this theme, the participant continued by recounting that the date of the stroke corresponds to the first anniversary of the son's suicide, that this event was emotionally charged, because he was not allowed to attend the celebrations that were forbidden to him by his ex-wife (the mother of his son).

This kind of comment, this apparently senseless logic between what is said and what seems to be understood by the participant, is not exceptional; we find it in most of the interviews of our research projects. He says the essential of a conflicting content that disturbs him at the highest level, but he talks about it as if he didn't know anything about it. We immediately see that we are dealing here with a struggle between a motion that the individual is trying to suppress and a management attempt that keeps the motion at a preconscious level. These are the effects of an unsuccessful use of defence mechanisms. We are talking here about an *ambivalent defence* in the form of denial. This case, this discursive logic, would require particular attention, which alone would deserve a discussion worthy of a publication of a specialized article. But isn't the same true of the nine participants who were part of the sample in our first pilot study?

Indeed, as soon as we give the floor to the circumstances surrounding a stroke, we are faced with some of the most relevant, if not phenomenal, content. Another attitude noted in our pilot study indicated a distinct and equally interesting logical structure. Here, the ambivalent opposition is not internalized by the person, but manifests itself between the individual and the discourse of those around him. He is a man met following

---

23. Circumstance: *circumstare; circum*: around; *stare*; what is standing.
24. This negative form, as an interview strategy, preserves the individual's defenses without confronting them. On the contrary, this type of discourse reinforces the subject and allows topics to be addressed without undermining the ambivalence of its defensive balance.

two transient ischemic attacks (TIAs) and a stroke that occurred in the same year, all three on the birthday date of his three stepsons. What is particular here is the fact that it is not the individual himself who informs us of the circumstances of stroke, but his spouse (the mother of his three stepsons) who was present at the interview. She tells us in an ironic tone: "He systematically has a stroke on their birthday, as if he was doing it on purpose to stop me from visiting them on that day." Later in the interview, by discussing with the participant, we will learn the conflictual emotional context of his new family situation. He had recently become a widower following tragic events and had met his new wife who already had three sons. These sons have always violently rejected him, refusing their mother's new union and marriage and even to be in the presence of this new stepfather. Stroke thus prevents, as the wife said, her from visiting her sons.

We immediately see that stroke seems to have a direct influence on the life situation of this family members (at least from what was said during the interview). We will have to return to the fundamental question of the benefits, advantages or disadvantages of stroke; as if stroke was able to accomplish, in the individual's place, what the individual is not consciously able to assume, achieve or decide.

Many examples of a parallel conception acting in the expression of stroke are widely disseminated by the media when we learn that *this* public figure has had a stroke: the day this musician gave his farewell concert, the day of the election when this politician ran as a candidate, the day this business leader began appearing in court, the day of a very important deadline or the anniversary of an event (happy or tragic, birth or death) symbolically representative for this individual. On the other hand, as soon as we discuss the circumstances surrounding the occurrence of stroke in a public forum, we are immediately bombarded with specific details illustrating how an immediate family member or loved one has had a stroke under conditions that appear to be most significant to that person (dates, circumstances or events that are especially meaningful).

Let us note also the opposite, but equally popular attitude, which opposes (sometimes violently) any incursion of meaning, other than medical, when it comes to discussing pathological manifestations; stipulating that what is the disease is of a purely biological order (a form of genetic *act of God*), associating our kind of approach with mystical, far-fetched research, brushing astrology or numerology and without real interests. Thus, the subject is closed, gagged, all speeches becoming superfluous.

While these popular conceptions do not really advance debate, our studies and research projects provide us with the opportunity to move forward in exploring the understanding of the stroke universe, while allowing stakeholders to be in a better position to hear the specific issues of its phenopathological organization and to use a new methodology to investigate, prevent or clinically intervene.

PLEAD IN HIS/HER DEFENSE

The majority of participants invited to speak during an interview felt, in a certain sense and at various levels of intensity, called to the stand, called to testify. Many felt the need to plead their case, answering an implied question "What do you have to say for your defense?" A defence is thus understood, to varying degrees, as inherent to the speaking process, which may sometimes inhibit the course and conduct of the speech or have very little effect on it.

One of the interviewer's first tasks was therefore to reassure the participants and assure them of the independence of the process (external to government authorities, the health system and the quantity or quality of care received by health institutions). The interviewer had to guarantee the protection of data, anonymity and confidentiality of the comments collected, so that the interview took place in a climate of trust, an informal atmosphere, without any accountability or follow-up. It was also to promote free or indirect associations, to clarify that the interview did not seek to find any cause, reason or responsibility, that the questions remained open to dialogue, without seeking good or bad answers, without having anything to confirm or measure, to try to discover together situations or circumstances, links, coincidences or events, sometimes external, anecdotal or surprising, that could be associated with stroke.

Despite these indirect directions and instructions from the interviewer, we had to face more or less organized forms of defensive mechanisms. In addition to the two examples of the first form of *ambivalent defence* just mentioned, we had to deal with more radical mechanisms that greatly complicated the interviewer's task. Without making an exhaustive inventory of them, let us try to identify their main structure of expression.

Let us immediately say that several of the 37 participants in the study sample spoke in "good faith", respecting the instructions of the interview and submitting to the rules of the interview, despite their specific defense mechanism, inherent to their personality. However, some reluctant, recalcitrant participants had resistance that was difficult to circumvent (although they had nevertheless agreed, despite this and for different reasons, to participate in the study). Among these rebel defence structures, there is a second form of radical *folding* and strong *denial* that interacts from *external constraints*, causing the individual to speak reluctantly, wanting to say nothing compromising, as if he/she was talking under surveillance or had a huge secret to hide. In this defensive category, we find a member of a criminal motorcycle group or corrupt criminal organization, a drug dealer or tax evader who did not seem to appreciate receiving the interviewer's visit to their home (they probably agreed to participate in the study, wrongly believing that a refusal on their part could have attracted the attention of the health professional mandated to screen potential participants for our project).

Still in this defensive category, we were surprised to see, from such a small sample, the number of participants who received a *financial benefit* as a result of the stroke. Obtaining a lifetime disability pension or insurance premium, permanent participation in the social welfare assistance program, secondary benefits granted or grant programs obtained (as a result of stroke) to meet the needs of an immediate disabled family member appeared to be privileges directly associated with the diagnosis of stroke, long sought by the recipient. One participant (who probably lowered his guard during the interview) told us about the complexity of the procedures before he finally managed to meet with a physician known to sign disability certificates without question. Others have openly admitted that stroke (after several other unsuccessful attempts) has finally succeeded in ensuring that the person can leave an unbearable job (while providing them with enough income to survive).

It should be noted that only the informal context of the interview setting was favourable and conducive to obtaining such confessions. Despite a seemingly concrete defense mechanism, the interviews were successful, revealing results that were highly relevant to document the study. However, some information that would certainly have been very productive for knowledge transfer activities about stroke could not be addressed. For example, an individual who identified his spouse as a simple roommate, in order not to be penalized on the amount of his social welfare assistance program, refused to elaborate on the latter's involvement and role in the particular circumstances surrounding his stroke (involvement that seemed at first sight to be most decisive).

A third form of defence presents an *erratic*, even *uninhibited* discourse, pulling in all directions, sowing in all winds, to try to drown the fish. This discourse, scattered with inconsistencies and anachronisms, is very difficult to follow, flooding the interview space with information that is sometimes superfluous, aberrant or contradictory, mixing eras, staging an innumerable number of characters (often reversing their first names), making no effort for the interviewer to find his/her way around, making it impossible (on the spot) to reproduce any logical framework from the story. This form of defence is often used again when the circumstances surrounding the stroke seem obvious (or following revealing lapses), as if, feeling caught at the word, once the essential is addressed and blatant, all that remains is for the participant to try to create confusion, the ultimate attempt to get out of the game.

Although this latter form of defence had apparent similarities, or produced the same kind of discourse, it should not be confused with what we might call a *watered defence*, that is, a discourse produced by addiction, or even alcohol or drug intoxication, a habit that inhibits or disinhibits the conduct of the interview. Again, we were surprised to meet many participants who admitted to having a problem with alcohol or certain drugs (or to having been intoxicated at the time of the stroke). It is not surprising that the interview time is contaminated by the participant's addiction and that some seemed to be on hangover when the interviewer was met[25].

Another form of defence that may seem apparent, although it is totally distinct in terms of the personality traits involved, is that of *psychotic discourse*. One participant spoke openly about his acute psychotic episodes (which cannot be separated from the themes surrounding the onset of stroke); another reported hallucinations, while others talked about their use of neuroleptic or psychotropic medications. This discourse, these defences, leading the individual not to have the same reality test, meant that the comments collected required very particular attention during the analysis of the interviews.

---

25. Although some participants – claiming to be members of anonymous alcohol or drug groups and insisting that they had stopped using alcohol or drugs – tried to hide their regular use of alcohol or drugs, some details of the daily routine told during the interview (going to bars, breweries or lively parties with friends) as well as physical clues (such as the presence of several empty or full bottles in the individual's home) easily allowed the interviewer to detect their daily dependence. It should also be noted that some repetitive behaviours or strange attitudes of participants during the interview (tics, automatisms, mania, nervous laughter, coughs or spasmodic crying) may indicate to the interviewer that he/she is touching an area of ambivalence that is at the heart of the individual's defense mechanisms (we noticed, during the interviews, that one of the participants changed voice timbre when she was addressing contentious content).

A final form of defence is described as an *offensive defence* (which can become violent) that we have observed in individuals with strong repressed (ambivalent) components and a well-organized psychological conflict. Here, it is imperative for the individual not to submit to the rules of the interview, which has become a final struggle for his/her defence. He/she does not seem to be taken at his/her word, but trapped; he/she does not shoot in all directions, but with red balls on the messenger (in this case the interviewer and the threat he/she may represent). According to one participant with this form of defence, stroke does not need to be questioned, it is a genetic fatality, like cancer, and no other incidence of any kind can be considered. Systematically refusing to answer the interview, he will invariably deny all questions related to his experience, using more than 150 times the word "no" and 35 times the word "nothing" in an interview of less than one hour. Going after the interviewer, questioning his competence, training and methodology, he will ridicule the process, making very disparaging allusions. Despite this unbridled attitude and tone, the interviewer was able to calm the situation and obtain, using the data and information collected at the beginning of the meeting, interview content that will document a complex, well-developed and exemplary scenario about the circumstances that were particularly critical to the occurrence of stroke.

Forms of defence:

1. *Ambivalent* (internalized) defence in the form of denial
   1.b. Ambivalent opposition between the individual and the discourse of those around him

2. Defense by radical *folding* and strong *denial* that interact from *external constraints*
   2.b. The constraint conceals a *pecuniary advantage*

3. Defense by *erratic* or even *uninhibited* discourse
   3.b. *Watered* defense
   3.c. Defending a *psychotic* discourse

4. *Offensive* defence

PART 3

SIMILAR SIGNIFIER THEMES EMERGING IN SEVERAL INDIVIDUALS

This section presents the main themes common to several participants that emerged as meaningful and spontaneously associated with the onset of stroke. However, we begin with a brief description of the sample characteristics, taking care to present only the central trends, to ensure that the confidentiality of participants is maintained. Note that we are changing the order of presentation and the numbering of the case histories to each of the contents (or grouping themes) in order to make it impossible to identify the participants. No overlap, other than that due to chance, can therefore be made between the presentation orders and the numberings of the participants. The letter *P* refers to the participant's verbatim while the letter *I* corresponds to the interviewer's verbatim[26].

CHARACTERISTICS OF STUDY PARTICIPANTS

In order to collect data from at least 30 participants, 45 individuals were screened by the research nurse. Of these 45 individuals, two were only available on weekends, four could not be reached within the eight-week post-stroke period, one was excluded because he could not express himself clearly in French, and another was excluded following the interview due to a technical recording problem. These eight individuals were all men. We therefore conducted 37 interviews for which, on ten occasions, a relative was present, the majority of them the spouse (8/10), while

---

26. It should be noted that the discourse was spoken, recorded and transcribed, which unfortunately gives, in the case of reading, to lexical and syntactical errors. All verbatim were translated and double checked for accuracy by fully bilingual individuals.

in the other two situations, it was the presence of a son and the participant's mother. Participants were aged between 27 to 68 years with an average age of 56.3 ± 11.9 years and a proportion of 40.5% women (15/37). Participants were diverse in both side of stroke and stroke type (see Table 3.1) based on the TOAST classification (Adams et al., 1993).

TABLE 3.1

Participants' characteristics

	N=37
Age (mean ± standard deviation [range])	56.3 ±11.9 [27-68]
Gender	N (%)
– Women	15 (40.5)
– Men	22 (59.5)
Type of stroke	
– Ischemic	36 (97.3)
– Hemorrhagic	1 (2.7)
TOAST Classification	
– Small vessel occlusion (lacunar)	3 (8.1)
– Large artery atherosclerosis	7 (18.9)
– Cardio embolism	9 (24.3)
– Stroke of other determined aetiology	5 (13.5)
– Stroke of undetermined aetiology	13 (35.2)
Side of stroke	
– Right	19 (52.8)
– Left	16 (44.4)
– Bilateral	1 (2.8)
– Missing data	1
Type of residence	
– Owner	16 (43.2)
– Tenant	18 (48.6)
– Room rental	1 (2.7)
– Residence for autonomous persons	2 (5.4)
Living arrangements	
– Alone	11 (29.7)
– With spouse	13 (35.1)
– With children	4 (10.8)
– With spouse and children	8 (21.6)
– Other	1 (2.7)

Education level		
– High school	20 (54.1)	
– College	6 (16.2)	
– University	11 (29.7)	
Main occupation	Pre-stroke	Post-stroke
– Convalescence	0	13 (35.1)
– Work	18 (48.6)	6 (16.2)
– Housework	2 (5.4)	1 (2.7)
– Studies	1 (2.7)	1 (2.7)
– Retirement	10 (27.0)	10 (27.0)
– Non-employee/job search	1 (2.7)	1 (2.7)
– Social welfare	3 (8.1)	2 (5.4)
– Others	2 (5.4)	3 (8.1)

MAIN THEMES

The main theme, forming a kind of umbrella, encompassing and making it possible to make the link between each of the case stories, is interpersonal relationships. Indeed, in each of the stories told, participants spoke of a particularly meaningful relationship, tinged with ambivalence or lack of transparency, characterized by emotional overinvestment. The types of relationships mentioned were those with spouses, children, parents or siblings. For some, this relationship was particularly evident at a birthday or anniversary: "I'm less interested [in my birthday] as I think about my mother that day, she gave birth to me, that day I'll think about her. But I'm going to think of her, not me. It's not because I was born, it doesn't really matter that much" (P39)[27]. For others, it was about the relationship with a child or parent: "But this [her daughter's leaving home] didn't last long. She [daughter] came back after 6 months. Ah, she was fine with Mom, she said: ah, I'm changing my mind. I said: eh, mom, eh, it's beautiful, it's fun mom (laughs). She says: I'm never going to leave… I don't believe her. She will leave, but not under the same conditions" (P24). In some cases, the relational conflict was clearly stated, while in others, the conflict emerged through the interview, during the exchange, but was not necessarily consciously acknowledged by the participant. The events and circumstances specific to each participant contributed to emo-

---

27. In this section, the participant number refers to the order of screening by the research nurse, from 1 to 45 for 37 interviews.

tional overinvestment, especially "on that day", when the stroke occurred.

Birthdays and anniversaries

The birthday is certainly not a trivial day in an individual's year. This is a meaningful and symbolic date when encounters and relationships often occur, which can be characterized by emotional overinvestment. This birthday theme (including anniversaries) emerged as a meaningful element for 27 of the 37 participants (73%). For some, it was their own birthday. The importance of this anniversary, as a potentially stressful circumstance and with an increased risk of stroke of nearly 30% on its birthday, has already been identified as significant in a large epidemiological study (Saposnik et al., 2006). However, for other participants, the anniversary also emerged as a meaningful theme, but it was the birthday of a loved one (spouse, children, parent or sibling), the anniversary of marriage, the anniversary of the death of a meaningful person or a meaningful historical event (for example, the 10th anniversary of the World Trade Center attacks, an anniversary that occurred during our recruitment period). Some anniversaries, such as Valentine's Day or Christmas, were also recurring themes in the participants' discourses. Thus, the stroke date becomes a relevant entry point for opening a space for exchange during the interview about individually determining signifiers, or for introspection into the meaning of this date, or this time of year, for the person themselves.

Listening to one of the participants who had a stroke on her birthday (P19), one wonders if the stroke, precisely on that day, was not premeditated. Indeed, the day before her stroke, she had announced to her co-workers that the next day she would be absent by referring to the time of her birth:

> It happened on my birthday... it was funny, anyway. I: What do you usually do at your birthday? P: At my birthday, uh, you know, I work, if it's the week, I never take a holiday... There was a surprise party, he [spouse] had prepared it for Saturday with 40–50 people... I suspected it. I suspected that. But uh... I wasn't sure. You know, I was going fishing a little bit there... They all blew it, they all said, you're sick, it doesn't make sense.... These are guys from the office, then one came to see me, he was captivated because he said, I want you to tell me, you knew it was going to happen to you, because you joked about it, you told me, I said guys, tomorrow, 3:00 am it's over for me. Because I was born at 3:00 a.m.

Another participant (P11) was bedridden on his birthday, not because of stroke, but because of a severe flu. The particularity here is that the participant and his spouse insist on the exemplary state of health of the gentleman, who is never ill. His last big flu was 7 years ago, when his niece was born. His wife remembers because she was supposed to go help her sister and hadn't gone to take care of him. On his birthday, he had a bad flu that had put him to bed: "Because on weekends it was a weekend, my birthday was a Saturday. Saturday and Sunday, I spent the day in bed." During the interview, it was mentioned that the gentleman could not afford to be too sick because his health insurance card had recently expired, since his birthday: "No, but I had never been hospitalized... Spouse: But the worst thing is that the day before, he received his card because he is late in getting his health insurance card. He received it on Monday evening. He said: Now I can be sick. The next day he had his stroke (laughs). "

The date of stroke is for many people associated with a meaningful anniversary date. This date is anchored in the memory of the individual since there is a "coincidence" with this anniversary. But is that a coincidence? The participants' discourses maintain that there is no question of chance or coincidence. The famous "it's a Sunday. Sunday, I remember it very well, because it was my niece's birthday. I am her godmother" (P37) is not trivial. Indeed, for this person, the theme of motherhood and the relationship with her mother, the recent death of her mother and herself in an ambivalent role as a mother on a daily basis, but without having children, turned out to be omnipresent themes throughout the interview. She considers her niece precisely as her daughter: "Sure, I would have liked to have had children, because... But, I had children in a certain sense, because... my nephews, my nieces there, I always took care of them as if they were my children."

For another participant (P2), stroke occurred on the anniversary of her ex-spouse's death: "They [her children] didn't find her funny... No, they lost their father too. No, they didn't think it was funny... it was the anniversary of my husband's death. (laughs)... they said that's no fun, what's happening to that darn date... We're going to delete it from the calendar! (laughs)." In addition, for one participant (P43), stroke occurred on the first anniversary of the sale of his company: "I sold my business, so... yes, yes. It's been a year, it's been sold, I think.... Yes" while during the interview, there were references to past conflicts with former partners: "I had partners and it wasn't always good. Besides, I lost a thirty-year-old friend, because he started stealing from me, so... no." Elsewhere, during the interview, he mentions: "[...] it has nothing to do with stroke, but I was going to... The week the stroke came along, I was going to invest in a new business [with a new partner], so I lost that opportunity."

For other participants, the overinvested relationship is the one with the spouse, and stroke occurs precisely on the anniversary of the marriage, the spouse's birthday or Valentine's Day (which symbolizes for them the celebration of lovers). For example, for this participant (P30), stroke occurs when all the preparations for *a romantic trip* are completed: "So we said to ourselves: and it goes well, we're going to be in love, in the South, in the sun, for our anniversary. It was our 13th anniversary together." Another participant (P38) reported that his stroke occurred on his wedding anniversary date. His wife corrected him by reminding him that he suffered it not the same day, but a few days before his first wedding anniversary: "Spouse: A year ago, we were supposed to go celebrate, and he was in the hospital. P: That's it." During the interview, the gentleman reports having already suffered a heart attack about 20 years ago, while dancing at a friend's wedding and his ex-wife had just left him a few months earlier to start a new life with one of the couple's good friends. Indeed, for this individual, the theme of marriage emerges as a meaningful theme, emotionally overinvested, throughout the interview. P36 had a stroke a few days before his wife's birthday: "I: It was your birthday? Wasn't he there at your birthday? Spouse: No, no, we were in the hospital, we celebrated in the hospital (laughs)", while for P45, the stroke occurred the day before: "Yes. It was his [his spouse's] birthday. I: The next day? P: Yes. Nice gift." In the case of P34, stroke occurs on Valentine's Day weekend as the ambiguous subject of the circumstances of his separation emerges during the exchange: "Ah, why am I talking about this, I hate this [circumstances of his separation]. I: Well, it's just, it came up on the subject, I told you it might not be fun. I said we'd talk about all kinds of topics. P: Well, yes, it's that this case, it brings me back here, that's it. Make sure that's what it is... I: It's important to talk about it. No? P: Yes, well, yes. I: Is it a big deal? P: Yes, because I never mentioned it." A scenario with some similarities was also told by another participant (P35) who also had a stroke on Valentine's Day weekend (during a show), while the relationship with his spouse and ex-spouse was a recurring theme during the interview. He had bought tickets for a show scheduled for the Valentine's weekend and gave them to his current spouse for Christmas: "Yes. Valentine's Day, which we always celebrate... Oh yes. For us, it is very important."

Another important and meaningful period for many participants is Christmas and the holiday season. For one participant in particular (P26) who had a stroke in early January, the holiday season is a kind of family trauma. She recounts the conflict between her father and her family that occurred during the holiday season when she was a baby: "And at one point my father was shocked because he had a big snowstorm and didn't want to go. And my grandmother called him crying, calling him all the names, and we went anyway, we took the field [accident]. And he [father] was very scared, we never reached our destination. My mother was pregnant of my brother, and I was very young." She also mentions the rivalry with her 13-month-old younger brother and the presence of conflicts with her sister-in-law whom she met during this period: "It's not that she's a sister-in-law, it's that, her children are an accident. Yes, she and my brother were together not long ago, and she has a temperament that we all know my brother hated... he would never have stayed with a girl like that..." The holiday season is a time of year when family gatherings are often omnipresent. When this event intersects with other emotionally overloaded circumstances – for example, for this participant, the break-up with her spouse just before the holiday season, a spouse who strangely resembles, in many ways, her brother: "I: He is a little like your brother, deep down? P: Yes and no. Well, yes, in a way, it's true..." – The onset of stroke, especially during the holiday season, makes sense here.

Let us highlight one of the most interesting aspects related to the denial of the importance of the birthday or anniversary. Indeed, when we asked if there was a particular anniversary or event at the time of the stroke, a typical answer was: "When did it happen? I: Yes. P: No. I: At the end of August or early September there is nothing? P: No, at the beginning of September, it's my birthday" (P1). Another participant (P11) had a stroke the day before his birthday, but made no mention of it during the interview, despite being asked directly, as if he had repressed and forgotten the date of the stroke. We also found these omissions in other participants. Indeed, P25 (who also had a stroke on his birthday) responds in a similar way and has "forgotten" what happened at his birthday that year, but can still report the presence of tension between his children, who usually meet on that day:

> No, this month, no, I was born in mid-December. I: What did you do on your birthday this year? P: Usually, I used to have dinner here. I: With? P: Both. I: With whom? P: My son and my daughter. It was still being talked about, but, you know, it was tense, but it was still being talked about. I: For your birthday, they would come. P: Uh, yes. I: This year, what was planned? P: This year, was there anything planned for my birthday? Ah, we were going to dinner at the restaurant. I: With the two children? P: Yeah, with the two kids, I don't know, we didn't go, I don't know why. I don't remember that. I: You didn't go this year? P: No. I: What did you do at your birthday this year? P: I don't remember that. I: Don't you remember? P: No. I must have stayed here, I didn't do much special.

An eloquent example of the denial related to the importance and meaning of the anniversary date is P12. Here is an excerpt from the exchange where his birthday and the meaning of that date are discussed:

> It was my birthday two days before [the stroke]. Two days before that. We do nothing at my birthday... No, no, no, for me, my birthday is a number, and it ends there... My father died on my mother's birthday, my mother also died on her birthday. We're moving on to other things, yes. Because I'm moving on to other things before my birthday right now. It's my birthday today, but tomorrow is over. I don't know. I don't know. My birthday was never something I stopped at... if she [spouse] doesn't tell me, it's your birthday, well I'll come by without talking about it only... no. I used to smoke, but I quit when I was 40. It's been 28 years already. I: What made you stop? P: I was tired of smoking. I: You were tired? P: I just took the package and said: it's over. And it was over, yes. I: When was that? P: At forty years old. I: At your birthday? P: Yes. I: Nothing happens at your birthday, huh? (laughs) P: Yes, that's exactly what it is.

Thus, resistance can manifest itself as a denial, as in the example cited above, or as a minimization of the importance of the emotionally over-invested period. For example, P22 mentions: "No, there is no birthday, there is my sister who has her birthday at this time except that we were absent." He had his stroke in mid-December, between his sister's birthday and Christmas, and insists that, since his father's death, Christmas no longer has any meaning "for his mother". However, the interviewer did not ask him specifically about his relationship with his mother; it is the participant who continually talks about his mother throughout the interview:

> No, no, it's never been, and my mother has never, since my father died, it seems like Christmas for her it couldn't have any meaning... And one more thing, we see each other quite often. I think it's a little bit everyone, when it's small and close families, you see them quite often that Christmas is no longer an excuse to see each other. It's just, we celebrate it the same way normal, it's a meeting, you know, it's a chance to get together, but not... nothing special. It's not a big deal for the rest of us.

Later in the interview, the participant reported that this period also coincides with the first anniversary of his mother-in-law's death: "Died, uh, died in the past holiday season. It's been a year now."

Beyond denial and minimization, some resistance can be so strong that some participants went so far as to avoid mentioning completely that the stroke period was consistent with a meaningful anniversary for them. One participant (P29) avoids mentioning that the birth of her nephew, her brother's son, coincides exactly with the occurrence of her stroke, at the time of a family meeting, very common according to her: "I: Then, in this area, are there birthdays or, uh…? P: No. I: Nothing is happening… P: We are all, uh… at the end of May, beginning of June, otherwise uh… October to December. So… there is no… I: These are empty periods? P: Yeah, really empty (laughs)… Yeah, yeah, yeah, no, there's no… there's nothing special, there's nothing…" The interview, interspersed with nervous laughter, took place three months after the stroke and recounted the circumstances of the first symptoms of stroke: "Everyone sleeps there, then… then my brother too had a little baby, so… I : Oh yes ? P: Yeah, he had a baby three months ago."

Parenting

One type of relationship that emerged frankly and unequivocally for almost half of the participants (n = 18/37) was the relationship with their children. This relationship, which was spontaneously mentioned throughout the interview, was tinged with ambivalence or overinvestment. We had a few cases where the participant was a mother of a young child and for whom the onset of stroke had the effect of ending the idea of another pregnancy, which seemed to be pleasing. For example, P30 discusses the idea of getting pregnant again after a stroke: "[…] it's like an acceptance process because he [spouse] might have liked it to have another child. So, but I can't anymore. Because of the stroke." Elsewhere, P29 associates motherhood with a calculated risk: "But no, that's right, because it [pregnancy] wasn't completely planned, but it wasn't either, uh… I mean, it was a calculated risk, if you want… In a way, it was kind of a good thing, let's say it like that, then if I ever, uh… it's ok…" The ambivalence regarding the role of parent and the responsibilities that accompany this role are evoked by P30 when she approaches a trip: "It was the first time to say [during a trip] that we got away from our parenthood for a week… But it was really the first time that we escaped, as a couple, all alone, as lovers. So ah yes, it's a lot of good" and by P17 which, following the stroke, aims to prioritize time for her: "[…] I kind of understood for example that I had to take time for myself, I don't have the choice to do it. This was different before [the onset of stroke]. Before, it was the baby, always the baby, if he cried, I had to be there right away. But then I realized that he can cry for two minutes and it's not a big deal right now."

For these women, the onset of stroke has also resulted in additional assistance to care for the child or children. For example, for P17: "And there's a girlfriend who comes to help me during the days he [the spouse] works. Make sure I'm never alone in the house." The same discourse can be found for P29: "I was able to take care of her, but the first month I always had someone with me. So, if I was tired, I would go to bed and then the person would take care of her", who also uses stroke to stop breast-feeding: "I was breastfeeding her at first. When, when I had that [stroke], I stopped, I mean because… I: She was still breastfed at that time? P: Yes. Yeah. But I'd already tried the bottle a couple of times, then she did not receive that very well… But now she had no choice (laughs). "

For another older participant (P5), the theme of motherhood was also raised spontaneously and consistently throughout the interview. She had her stroke at a time when she had to make herself available for her daughter who was trying to *get pregnant*. Ambivalence about her daughter's potential pregnancy was addressed as follows: "So I might be a grand-mother… I wish… No, but I wish it didn't work [her daughter's pregnancy], you know, but I think, I can't do that to her… I can't… do that, you know…" Her own pregnancies and especially her childbirths, which she recounted in detail, represent for her striking and traumatic moments: "You know, I had a caesarean section. Besides that it's disgusting, it's disgusting because I never talked about it, but… uh they didn't give me enough liquid so that uh… it wasn't endurable. So that's it… That's our uh, our life… supposedly that I almost died." Other women with adult children also testified throughout the interview about an overinvested re-lationship with their child. For one of them (P41), the relationship was al-most symbiotic; the participant clearly identified herself with her daughter, described herself as *both being similar* and the occurrence of her health problems allowed for an increased connection with her daughter:

> She [her daughter] was in shock. A lot, a lot, she cried a lot, her too… But, after that, she was strong. She was with me. At the time of the stroke, she was… I: She was already close, but then she was even closer, I guess? P: Yes, yes, yes, yes. Even more… she's even more glued. She calls me, every day, from work, at her lunch hour: how are you, Mom, eating well? I: Didn't she do that as much before? P: No. Are you eating well, are you correct?

For another (P3), who has several children, the overinvested relation-ship was with one of her children who took up almost all of the exchange. She describes this son as a "rescue" and, when the interviewer points out that she talks a lot about him, she answers:

> He's a guy who's very endearing, and I almost lost him as a baby… I almost lost him, he had some kind of bronchiolitis… He was 2 years old. I almost lost him… yes, very close to me. He was leaving, he was coming to tell me: Mom, I'm going there, there. And then he was coming back, and so on. Very young, he has always been like that. And older… Even then… It stayed the

same. I'm not telling you I don't like other siblings. I: No, I know, that's not what we're saying, but you feel he's close. P: This one, yes, that's it.

She describes this son as her confidant:

And if I have to confide, I'll confide in my son... There are things I say to my son, and there are other things I don't say to my husband, that I can say to my son. You know, sometimes we can hide things, sometimes we can hide things from our husband. We don't have to say everything, you know. Not... It's not because I don't trust my husband or give him the secret, but there are things that can be said, and there are other things that can't be said. That's it, that's it. My son has always been like that, you know. When I want to talk, or let off steam, you know... I: You know he's there... P: I know he's there, you know, anytime.

Still from the perspective of parenthood, we have had other cases where parenting responsibilities have become more constraining at a time when the child, with a particular disability, requires constant supervision, especially as he/she approaches adulthood. One of the participants (P15) described her child as follows: "[...] she is an unpredictable child, you know. I thought to myself, ah, so what happens, will happen! [during a restaurant outing]. You know at some point we know how to, uh, react and think, but there's always stress in it... yes. There's the unexpected that... Yes. Sometimes that's not manageable..." This participant had her stroke a few days before her child's birthday and, as a result of the hospitalization, missed the first friends' party organized for the occasion, precisely that year:

[...] it's a child who has a lot of trouble socializing, it was the first time she accepted to invite friends, so... I was in the hospital, so I didn't think we had to cancel... Even if I, you know I didn't feel good not being there for her birthday it's for sure, we had been talking about it for so long, it can't be that I wasn't there for her birthday, Lord!

For these other participants, the entire interview also focuses on the theme of mentoring their child, who is also in transition to adulthood. They describe their daily life (P11) as follows: "[...] with his illnesses, it's rock 'n' roll sometimes... always the same routine, sometimes quarrels, we're like an old couple"; (P32): "[In addition to his disability] he's diabetic. He can't go far. That's it... so... I take all the responsibility since he was born, you don't have a vacation..." He has been withdrawing from his responsibilities since his stroke and is particularly angry with the health system. Indeed, he feels he is not getting the support he needs for his situation: "They [the workers in the system] put everything on their side, I'm sending them to the devil anyway. I'm not losing my time with them.... I'm fed up.... I won't start walking, using a walker, at their meetings." It is interesting to note here that the onset of stroke has, in one case, brought the child closer whose relationship was already overinvested, while in others, stroke has allowed a decrease in parenting responsibilities. In short, in all cases, stroke has had what we can call positive consequences, in the sense that these consequences have given some kind of permission for closer relationship or disinvestment in the relationship with the child.

Identification with one of their parents

For other participants (almost one-third, 11/37), it was the relationship with their parents that captured most of the discussion. Indeed, many identified with one of their parents to explain the onset of stroke as a kind of fatality: "I knew I had had a stroke... I had seen my father do this" (P4). This participant insists on distinguishing himself from his father by testifying to his father's exemplary life: "My father had not smoked for 30 years, no alcohol, and he always played a lot of sports", unlike his own daily life characterized by alcohol abuse. According to him, his addiction would come from his mother's side, from whom he says he is very close. He agrees with his father on one point: "And what he [father] said, it's true: you come into the world with the gene, and at some point, at some time, some date, whatever you do in life, it will bloom, it will come out. Whatever you did." In his case, the onset of stroke occurred a few days before his mother's birthday and wedding anniversaries. Indeed, he excludes his father from his discourse when he mentions his parents' wedding date: "And she [mother] got married in... [date of marriage]." In another case (P22), the participant has a very poor explanation for having a stroke because his mother has never had one: "Worse still, my mother has never had a stroke, she hasn't had one, she's 75 years old."

A few other participants dedicated the heart of the exchange to praising their mother: "Oh, I had a good mother, eh Lord. Everyone has good ones, I guess, but in any case, there are some that are better than others, huh? Yeah. Then my mother and I would spend several hours on the phone by, by day, by week..." (P6). P37, who also recently lost her mother (just like P6), says of her: "Well, yes, she was my mother, she was my friend, my confidant, my outings' friend, my mother she was everything to me. Everything. Everything. Oh, yeah, my mother, she was precious. Yes." This other participant (P9) clearly identifies with his mother. He describes her as an anthropologist with a free mind:

I: You don't need a lot of sleep, you seem to say? P: No. My, my mother was the same. My mother was exactly like that, she read until 2am in the morning, sometimes 3am, then… she went to bed, then she got up the next day. Do that, uh… it's genetic maybe… My mother… when she was young, she, what she really liked was geography, and she always stayed, uh… anthropologist, if I can say, uh…

When the interviewer asks him about his (obsessive) collection for an unusual object, he says: "I think it's more personal… that's like… it came to me, it came to me that it's, it's an anthropological connection. It's an anthropological object." In another case (P31), the stroke would have occurred at the same time of year and time of day as his mother's: "How it happened is that, it looks like she [mother] got up during the day. And then she was weird, she took a shower… it's because she doesn't feel good, and she says funny things, she went to bed, it took a whole day. Then in the evening… they took her to the clinic… And then, at the end of the day, the next day, well, it looks like a stroke after all…" He then recounts the circumstances of his stroke: "I woke up in the morning as usual… got up, got dressed, came to get my coffee… Well, I went to the bathroom to take a shower, to blow my nose and it was when I took the handkerchief that I found my hand strange. But I didn't think I had anything. After that, I think I went to bed, it's a black out, because I don't remember what I did." It should be noted that this participant did not make an explicit link during the interview regarding the blatant similarity of the circumstances of his stroke with the one of his mother. On another note, this other participant (P6) demonstrates an openness to the possibility that his emotionally over-invested relationship with his mother may have any impact on his health problems:

> But that's, that's, that's… I don't think it has anything to do with that… I'm sure it has no relation with that… I mean, it comes from far away… but let's say sorrow like that [his mother's death] we don't often… I've seen several people die, my father, it also made me feel… From that moment on, my dear, from the moment my mother, uh my mother became seriously ill… My diabetes… went up and stayed high. No way to get that down again. No way to get that down again. Is that related? I don't know that. Maybe yes, emotions do make a difference, it's true that there are many things that influence life right now. But uh….

Finally, this participant (P28), who identifies herself with her mother, says she is surprised to have had a stroke. In fact, she was convinced that she would never have a stroke, but that she would suddenly die, like the rest of her family on her mother's side: "First, I never thought I would have had a stroke. It's crazy, huh? I never, ever, ever, me, it was, I'm going to die all of a sudden. Me, because that's the way my mother's whole family is. Everyone, either by going to bed, by sitting on the toilet, it's always been." Her mother died suddenly from the heart while watching a movie. Ten years after her mother's death, this participant retires and begins to have heart problems. She describes the onset of the first symptoms of her stroke as follows:

> I sit down to watch TV, ah, well, I said, it's happening again. And I say: ah, I don't need it, all that, I felt it here, it starts there, ah well. Ah, my Lord. But I didn't think it was for all of a sudden, black in front of me. I: Did you think it was still the discomfort as you had already had several times that came back often? P: Yes, yes, yes. That's what it was like. But then when I had the dark, seeing black, I told myself: oh, no, no, no, it was no more fun. Then, I left and went to bed in bed right away. I went to lie down in bed…

This section shows that the relationship with a parent, even if the parent is deceased, can have such a meaningful individual significance that it takes up almost all of the exchange, which focused on the circumstances surrounding the trigger of stroke (if it is appropriate to recall). It should be noted that the importance of this relationship is not necessarily consciously recognized by the participant, but it emerges in the discourse when a space is allowed. Indeed, even among participants who were reluctant to take the floor, the content of their speech was on a theme that was necessarily meaningful to them. For example, one participant (P22) spent a good part of the exchange denying, saying "no" 150 times in less than an hour, and despite this, he mentioned his "mother" more than 30 times without being invited to talk about her explicitly.

Addiction

Current or past excessive use of alcohol or drugs was another theme that emerged from our discussions in more than a third of the participants (14/37). This consumption took a significant place in the daily lives of these individuals, even for those who no longer consumed: "In alcoholics anonymous, there are anniversaries. Well, we celebrate, we celebrate anniversaries. And then I was stuck with my cake, because it was the day I took my cake [of abstinence]" (P10). Some participants' discourses were particularly characterized by a lack of transparency and honesty in their content. For example, one participant (P1) who reported that he had stopped drinking ten years earlier described his alcohol consumption as follows:

> I stopped completely… no, I stopped drinking about four years ago. I've been drinking nothing for two years now. I: You haven't taken anything, nothing for two years. P: Two years I can say I have a beer occasionally. I: When

there's a dinner party or at a party? P: Uh, Saturday we went... we had a bottle of wine for the two of us, so I had a glass or two, but here sometimes I have a beer I mean in a summer I had six bottles of beer... No, the bottles are there, I said there will always be some, there's beer in the fridge, there will always be some. I've never been uh, first I drank strong drink, but lastly it was beer and wine. But there will always be [beer in the fridge].

Let us note a similarity in the discourse of this participant (P2) regarding her alcohol consumption: "I take some, I don't take alcohol... No, I've never taken some... from time to time, in the summer, when it's very hot on weekends, let's say I'll have a beer. But it's not uh... And it's not every day, it wasn't every day, I'm not a drinker uh, no, I've never been brought up to it..." (note that it was obvious that this participant lived in an environment conducive to drug and alcohol abuse). There is clearly a tendency among some participants to minimize their consumption: "I had taken a couple of beers... I: But when you take a couple of beers, is it really a couple of beers, or is it until falling? P: Until the blackout" (P4).

In addition, other participants mentioned their drug use without any censorship and from the outset. For example, this participant (P42) recounted, at the beginning of the interview, the circumstances of her stroke: "We were sitting talking with friends, and I had just used. I: Used what? P: Cannabis. Yes. And that's it, that's it. I thought it was my, my joint that was working. Yes, yes, yes. I thought it was my joint that was working, but I always fell on my left side. All the time. I couldn't sit up straight like that because I was falling." Another participant (P17) described it this way: "I always smoke a joint from time to time, but it's, say, when I need to sleep. Because I'm not a person who sleeps easily. If I smoke a little joint, I know that in the next 5 minutes... I: You'll fall asleep. P: Well, that's right. It helps me for this." In the same vein, one participant (P13) mentioned: "I have been taking drugs since I was 18 years old." This is also the case with this one (P9): "I have smoked, uh... all my life... cannabis... Since the stroke I almost stopped taking it. Uh... I smoked cannabis for 40 years".

Indeed, the occurrence of stroke would act, at least in the first few months, as a source of motivation for some people to stop consuming, in order to meet the social imperatives of good health while ensuring that a possible recurrence is prevented. This participant's discourse (P8) illustrates well the tone also found in many other individuals:

Well, at that time, I was drinking a lot... Since the stroke, not a drop!... I don't even have a desire or interest. Even when my son comes here sometimes, has a glass of wine and he says, does it bother you that I drink in front of you? Pfft, you can drink as much as you want, I don't mind. Well, I think that, in any case, the impression I have is that drinking, being stressed, uh, smoking, we won't deny this, it can be causes... Well, there I cut that, the next step will be to cut the cigarette! Uh, it can, in any case, help prevent us from not having more.

This other participant (P11) presented a similar discourse, but related to smoking: "In the beginning, after I got out of the hospital, I was always scared... I was smoking, except I wasn't swallowing the smoke... And then after that it fell down again... it lasted maybe 3 weeks... about 3 weeks, 1 month. You know, but... I'm not breathing it. There's always a little bit of it coming in, but... it's not as bad because right now... I was taking a puff, I was taking it, I was blowing it out. Like when I was a kid."

In short, alcohol or drug use was an important and meaningful theme for many of the participants, even among those who had stopped consuming for several years. Heavy drinkers in particular represented a challenge for the interviewer. Indeed, their speech was particularly defensive, evasive or simply contradictory, as if they had something to hide. Paradoxically, this style has not been found among users of soft drugs.

Being sick as a secondary benefit

Of all the themes common to several participants, the one that is applicable to all without exception is undoubtedly a positive appreciation of the consequences of stroke. This may seem surprising at first glance, since the occurrence of a stroke is usually conveyed as a misfortune, a disaster, or even a catastrophe. Without detracting from the tragedy associated with a health problem as important as stroke can be, its occurrence at this particular time has made it possible for some to avoid a highly meaningful and emotionally overloaded activity, such as a birthday, an anniversary or a planned event such as a trip or authorized a work leave. Indeed, as the verbatim presented in the previous pages have shown, the onset of stroke has enabled many to avoid a meaningful anniversary, birthday or event that was planned in the days that followed. For others, stroke allowed a work leave when their working context was, in these cases, ubiquitous during the interview and expressed as a source of constraint. For example, P33's wife expresses herself this way about her spouse's work: "But I think that the fact that he was no longer able, but disgusted to work, with the sweat of his brow in the summer." And then the gentleman goes on: "Ah, I was really disgusted... I: Does it suit you a little bit to be off work? P: Yes, yes, yes. Ah, I'm happy now." In another case (P8), the constraint to work is clearly related to a relational conflict: "At the time, what stressed me was the, at work, because I work with someone who is completely opposite to me, and uh I often work with him, so it doesn't make for a work atmosphere that is very much fun... and then, well, I can say that I have trouble dealing with that." However, it appears that the individual in question is in early retirement and was only working three days a week, whereas after the stroke this participant benefited from a gradual return to work of two days a week, precisely the two days during which the individual he cannot tolerate does not work. These excerpts clearly express the consequences of stroke, which we can easily label as positive.

For others, stroke has put them in a state of illness that consolidates a disability status associated with a financial benefit. Indeed, for example, this participant (P4) is very happy to have been able, thanks to stroke, to confirm his status as a disabled person:

> Well, the income is... It's average. Well, now they're giving me the full price on welfare... Since I'm unfit, because the doctor signed me as unfit... yes. The doctor signed off as unfit for life. For life. I: Is it a [doctor] you know well? P: No, it was my cardiologist who sent me there, because by dint of saying: my feet hurt, my legs hurt, she said: she sent me to see that doctor, he finds the most bizarre sores in the world.

Finally, in some cases, this status of being ill has legitimized the disempowerment of parenting or increased the proximity of the relationship to an emotionally overinvested relative. A mother (P17) thus approaches the decline in her responsibilities towards her child: "And it's sad because he's so happy all the time, this little baby smiles all the time, he wakes up at 4 am in the morning, big smile, you know." Another mother of adult children (P2) was able, thanks to stroke and her new status as a sick person, to both reduce her responsibilities and favour reconciliation. She says that now, as a result of stroke, there is no longer any question of her children returning home, whereas before stroke: "You know when they leave home too quickly, they often come back. I: They're coming back, huh? P: Well, they took turns doing it! I: Oh, yeah? P: Oh yes! (laughs)" and thus refers to her post-stroke relationship with them: "[the children] are closer and they call me more often... Yes, are more worried, yes. They call me more often, they come more often [but will never come back to live again at home]."

In short, this traditional qualitative analysis of verbatim highlighted some themes common to several participants. The main theme, encompassing all, is unequivocally that of interpersonal relationships. These are current relationships with a spouse, child or parent, and sometimes past relationships with a person who is now deceased, in most cases mother or father. These relationships are sometimes emotionally overinvested or characterized by ambivalence and a form of mandatory subsidiary responsibility. In all cases, however, the onset of stroke necessarily changed what was expected in their daily lives. Indeed, listening to participants talk about stroke, it is clear that the timing of the event is not trivial. The next part presents precisely the details of these events and circumstances, anchored in a phenoanalytical analysis.

PART 4

MAIN CIRCUMSTANTIAL THEMES OF THE STROKE

ANALYSIS PRESENTATION

It should be noted at the outset that we are faced with a major ethical problem in the subsequent analysis and further development of the content of the case histories of the study participants, namely the need to respect confidentiality. It would have been ideal to present in a single draft the signifiers, events and circumstances surrounding the stroke of the project participants; this would have allowed us to express in full clarity all the relevance and phenomenological rigour of our analyses, but we could not proceed in this way. It is clear that this respect for confidentiality causes us to lose some of the dynamics that occur in each case history – nothing is more true than the very thing – but we still believe that we have succeeded in preserving the essential meanings of the mechanisms that are perceived as triggers of stroke.

This is why we divide the presentation of the contents into seven distinct spaces defined by the logic of the theoretical framework that structures the analysis. As mentioned above, we are changing the order of presentation and, if necessary, the numbering of the case histories to each of the contents (or grouping themes), so as to make it impossible to identify the participants. So we present: 1) the dates and events when the signifiers (*Objekt*) manifest themselves; 2) the particular meanings of this event for the individual at the time it occurs (first reduction); 3) the aggravating circumstances that this event causes and brings back to the core of the individual's attempts at suppression and repression (second reduction); 4) the *Gegenstände* to which the participants refer; 5) the phenogenetic substrates of the inherited pathological predispositions of the individual and his/her family; 6) the physical sites where the first symptoms of stroke occurred; and 7) the effects, benefits and disadvantages, advantages and impediments caused by stroke. These seven spaces (or cluster themes) are presented in turn in chronological order by interview date, or by stroke date, and in alphabetical order by the name assigned to identify the case histories, or by the name of the central theme in question in the analysis.[28]

In order to preserve this confidentiality, we must omit specific personal details, hide or modify particular links that could potentially allow us to trace the same individual through the different parts of the presentation. If necessary, we use analogies or metaphors to express the logical organization of the theme without disclosing specific details or nominative information that could identify them. These analogies (or metaphors) may change at each of the seven grouping themes of the presentation.

It should also be noted that the content covered during the interviews – with the exception of socio-demographic data, personal information, stroke and hospitalization dates – was not known to hospital staff. As mentioned above, only the structural organization and informal context of the interview were conducive to providing us with access to such content. Finally, it should be noted that, in many cases, the subject him/herself is unaware that the meaning of the links identified in the interview content concerns him/her and, with the help of the amnesia of the defence mechanisms, cannot become aware that this is his/her own case. On the other hand, in previous publications concerning the disclosure of personal content, we have observed the opposite phenomenon, where several individuals wanted to inform us that they had identified themselves in the case histories and were convinced that these stories presented part of their private life when they were not at all involved.

ANALYSIS OF THE MAIN CIRCUMSTANTIAL THEMES OF THE STROKE

Spontaneously, when we hear about stroke, we hear essentially two levels of discourse: first, the person who has had the stroke tells what they think is the *external* cause(s) of their stroke (what we call their *Gegenstand*); second, health professionals and caring staff discuss the clinical characteristics and data of stroke (type, side, etiology, severity level, risk factors, care and rehabilitation plan, and so on). Is that what it means to talk about stroke?

If we do give the person who has had a stroke the opportunity to

---

28.   Note that spaces 1, 4, 5, 6 and 7 are presented in the form of a list.

speak, if we ask them to talk to us openly, free of clinical instructions, without any knowledge of the facts, outside a prescribed, rigid, established plan of care, we will quickly be surprised to find that the topics covered no longer have anything to do with what we were used to hearing, concerning the heart of the subject rather than his/her head. We will hear seemingly trivial, even anecdotal things outside the usual discourse. Far from being *external to* stroke, we will see that *these things* express the essence of the subject of stroke.

Stroke breaks out in its own time and space. It occurs on this date, in this environment and in this space which remain its specificities. As we wrote, stroke occurs on this date and in this place, in relation to an event that occurs vertically in front of the individual. If stroke becomes a phenomenon, it is because it actualizes, reminds, animates, reactivates or revives horizontally an emotional conflict that the consciousness cannot support, manage or take charge of. This morbid phenomenon is determined *a priori* by a genetic substrate that characterizes the type of disease; it is in the presence of a genetic heritage that is expressed in and by the person's immediate environment to fix his/her phenogenetic baggage.

By suspending our judgment (*épochè*) that stroke is an accident (*Gegenstand*) that occurs outside of an *intentional* structure – that is, subjective, meaningful and significant – here is what we hear by giving voice to stroke.

List of stroke *events* and *dates*

This is a chronological listing of the specific events that were mentioned by participants at the time of the stroke. It should be noted that these strokes took place over a seven-month period, between August 22nd, 2011 and March 28th, 2012.

Symbolic event (Φ)

The event corresponds to the date of a:

• All Saints' Day or All Souls' Day	• Halloween
• Anniversary or historical event	• Holiday season
• Candlemas	• New Year's Day
• Christmas	• Valentine's Day
• Death or anniversary death of a public figure	

Private event (-φ)

The event corresponds with a:

• A trivial event overloaded with meaning	• Life habit changes
• Anniversary or meaningful event	• Lifestyle change:
– (family or relative)	– Change in marital status, citizenship
– (self or meaningful person)	– New union, new cohabitation
• Birth	– Relocation, moving, exile
• Birthday	• Murder, suicide of a meaningful person
• Breakdown	• Retirement
• Death of a meaningful person	• Severe conflict (family relationship, professional)
• Departure, distancing of a meaningful person	• Show, cultural event or TV show (evoking a significant theme)
• End of relationship	
• Financial change	• Significant deadline
• Holidays	• Significant meeting
• Illness or treatment of a meaningful person	• Stroke of a meaningful person
• Illness or treatment of the subject	• Subject's Stroke Anniversary
• Important activity	• Trip, major travel
• Important appointment	• Wedding

Events surrounding the onset of stroke (Why that day?)

1st reduction, phenomenological reduction

Starting from a signifier, or *Objekt*, that frames stroke in space and time, various events are determined by aggravating circumstances that "trigger" stroke. Referring to the verbatim of the interviews, here is how the event can be emotionally overloaded by repressed content that recalls the circumstances that the conscience is trying to repress. Here, presented chronologically by interviewer meeting date, we find the various events surrounding the onset of stroke (note that two distinct events may condense, coincide and correspond to the same stroke or that the same individual may have had more than one stroke).[29]

[1] On the evening of his birthday dinner, things that cannot be heard, that cannot be said, were discussed by the lady who accompanied the individual (she was then intoxicated by alcohol). Mister insists on specifying that this lady, who seems to be the central character of his existence, is not his companion, despite the fact that she is a true copy of the woman of his life, from whom he separated 10 years ago. He denies any form of intimacy with this lady, claiming that she must be homosexual. The man with hearing problems no longer wears his hearing aid since that evening[30].

[2] The stroke occurred on the night of the tenth anniversary of his wife's murder, killed by her father to save the family's honour (this father could not stand his daughter's extramarital relationship). During that night, the man said he felt and relived, through the symptoms of his stroke, the armed attack that killed his ex-wife: leg pain (first shot) and chest pain (fatal blow to the upper body). In the year of the stroke, the man had recently been living with a new spouse strangely reminiscent of his deceased spouse, with the same beliefs and family pressure as the latter. The subject interprets the coincidence of dates as special, bizarre, random, claiming to not be superstitious. According to his wife, everything that happens is because of this anniversary date which is a fatality.

[3] The first symptoms of stroke reportedly appeared on the day of the death of a famous Canadian politician, when the death of this character, whom the lady held in high esteem, was announced. The stroke occurred during a trip when the woman was accompanied by her son. The lady says she is very attached to this son, who seems to be the most meaningful person in her social network. During this stay, there would have been confidences told to the son, the kind of confidences she wouldn't even tell her husband.

[4] This man's stroke occurred during the week of his mother's anniversaries (birthday and marriage anniversary) and birthdays of the two [only] people who are most meaningful to him. The individual was at the

---

29. In this sense, it should be recalled that 37 individuals participated in the study, but that we will report 39 events.

30. This was the first interview conducted for our study and served as a model for subsequent interviews, identifying areas for improvement. The participant was very reluctant to participate in the interview, the fact that the topic of confidentiality was at the centre of his concerns probably did not help things. The question of the individual's alcohol consumption was also very ambivalent and turned out to be a behaviour to be hidden (which increased the constraining intensity of the meeting with the interviewer).

gym at the time, in a training session. He knew exactly what was happening, having seen his father have the same thing and die from a stroke.

[5] This woman's stroke occurred at the time of her daughter's scheduled insemination, which she was supposed to attend. Despite her mother's stroke (and the fact that she will not be able to be present), the daughter's insemination will still take place. Associating, from experience, childbirth with a risk of death, the woman hopes that this insemination will have a negative result.

[6] A few months before the stroke occurred, the death of her mother, to whom the participant was very attached, triggered an uncontrollable increase in blood sugar levels, hence the desire to participate in diabetes research to test a new drug. The stroke occurred the night before the day this study began, when the individual was lying in his lazy-boy, with his arms on each side of his thighs. He spontaneously associates this position with the memory of the father's death, lying down, at rest, undergoing an electrocardiogram. Surrounding the date the stroke occurred, seven years earlier, the man had had six bypasses. Earlier that year, he was deeply disturbed by the death of his younger brother (heart problem) on their mother's birthday, the day before his own birthday.

[7] This man has a strong cardiopathic history, having suffered a heart attack, three bypasses and two strokes. He had his heart attack at the same age as his father had his heart attack, and his three bypasses were performed around the dates of his father's birthday and death. As for the two strokes, they occurred respectively on the departure dates abroad of the two persons meaningful to this individual: his son and his current spouse. Around these dates, there is also talk of confidences and a private meeting with the same son, an encounter during which the son informs his father of changes in his career choice and especially of his sexual orientation, homosexual. The fact that the participant is a radical homophobe and declares himself to be one complicates things and amplifies the emotional burden of this coming-out that deeply affects and disrupts him[31].

[8] Stroke occurred at a time when the individual was no longer able to be around and support a co-worker, a relationship that had become intolerable and caused severe pressure and arrhythmia for nearly two years. In recent years, he had taken many steps to end this relationship, filing two formal requests for reclassification with his employer, without obtaining

31. In the following section, we will have to come back to the consequences associated with the fight against the existence of homosexual components.

satisfaction. Only stroke made it possible to make his employer understand the seriousness of his demands.

[9] The stroke occurred on the weekend scheduled to formally initiate the move of the participant's youngest son (on the floor of the triplex where the individual, owner of the building, lived). His oldest son also lived in the building, next door to his brother's apartment. This move seemed a fateful event for the three individuals, an event overloaded with meaning that shattered the principle of trinity that had always united them. After the stroke, the oldest son will urgently take his father to hospital and then commit suicide.

[10] The first symptoms of stroke appeared in the morning as the participant waited for his brother to visit in the afternoon. This brother, who lived outside the region, visited him so that he could drive him to the airport (travel to Europe with his wife). That morning, the man wanted to run errands to greet his brother and prepare him a dinner, but stroke symptoms prevented him from remembering his personal identification number (PIN) to pay for his purchases. Panicked, ashamed and embarrassed, the individual cancelled his transaction. In addition, he was unable to drive his car to the airport, the couple had to travel to the airport by bus, subway and shuttle.

[11] The stroke occurred on October 31st, on Halloween. The participant pointed out that this Halloween evening was special because it would be the last time his son (who has an intellectual disability and is officially under the custody of the participant) would go out on the streets of the neighbourhood to collect sweets; indeed, in the following days, this son would reach his majority and would then, according to him and his father, be too old to *celebrate Halloween*. Later, during the interview, we learn that the legal age of the son is all the more meaningful, because it marks the end of the government's responsibility for the son. Living on social welfare and facing significant financial hardship, the individual does not know how he will now be able to meet his obligations. He relies on a disability pension and a babysitting allowance that could be granted to him because of the changes in his state of health that would be caused by his stroke.

[12] The stroke occurred on his birthday. The participant repeatedly insists that dates, especially birthday dates, especially his own, mean nothing to him ("it's only a number, it ends there"). Despite these statements, he notes that the birthday dates seem overloaded with associations in his family: his father died on his mother's birthday, his mother died on his

own father's birthday, the mother-in-law died on the individual's birthday, a few days before her own birthday. Still despite this insignificance, the participant added that he wanted to wait until his birthday to change his life habits and quit smoking.

[13] The attacks at the Word Trade Center in September 2001 had greatly disrupted this man, to the point of causing him a profound psychotic episode. He was then hospitalized and absolutely wants to forget this traumatic period of his life. Exactly 10 years after these events, the individual was scheduled for a psychiatric appointment to meet with his physician to monitor his condition. On the day of the appointment, he suffered suddenly from a severe emphysema attack, requiring hospitalization, and was unable to report to psychiatry. The appointment was postponed two months later. The stroke occurred on the day this second appointment was scheduled. At the time of the interview, more than three months later, he had not yet met his psychiatrist.

[14] Stroke had the effect of cancelling the couple's annual trip south to spend the winter season (a trip that the couple had systematically made for nearly 30 years). Towards the end of the interview, before leaving home, the interviewer learned surreptitiously that, the previous year, the daughter of the gentleman's best friend, considered like their own daughter, had visited them for a few weeks at their southern residence. Tragically, on her return to Montreal, she died in a car accident.

[15] This woman's stroke occurred on her daughter's 20th birthday (a girl with an intellectual disability, being very "difficult to live with"). To mark this event, the lady had planned a party at their home and, for the first time, had agreed to invite friends over. According to the lady, this long-prepared event was still very stressful, as it was impossible to predict her daughter's reactions. In addition, the age of 20 was significant because it represented the last year that her daughter will be able to attend the Day Centre, which had been caring for her daily since her early school years. The day after her daughter's birthday heralds an uncertain future and a step into the unknown.

[16] This stroke gives the appearance of a walk-the-talk; at the beginning of the interview, the woman discusses the theme of staging the particular events surrounding the occurrence of her stroke: living during the week in a home separate from her spouse (work requirement), she was alone in her apartment, she forgets the password on her cell phone that gives access to her contacts, forgets her spouse's phone number and forgets that she had turned off the ringing of her apartment phone during the

week. Anyway, she quickly realized that the stroke had temporarily caused her to lose her speech.

[17] At the beginning of the interview, the young woman, a mother of two children (a two-month-old baby and a two-year-old toddler), explains how the stroke gave her a break; now others are caring for her children. She sees only benefits in stroke: time for herself, she is never alone at home again, she gets help from a friend, mother and sister. She explains: "Basically, I only have four hours left to spend alone with the little ones, which is not dramatic, on that, the younger one sleeps two (which is very sad because this baby is always in a good mood)." She points out that before the stroke she was constantly alone at home with the children. She even had to take a taxi to the hospital alone when the stroke symptoms started. Finally, stroke was beneficial because it ended the possibility of having a third child (despite the spouse's desire). Through stroke, she was able to accomplish what she consciously did not dare to do.

[18] This individual who presents a *watered* and *erratic* defence does not mean anything clear or "incriminating" about the events surrounding his stroke; in fact, he speaks as if he were in a labyrinth. Despite this, the interview tells us that the scenario for this stroke revolves around the relationship with a significant woman: a colleague who was back at work on the evening of the stroke (after a prolonged absence). However, the man is unable to specify the terms of the relationship with this woman, if it is true that she was the one who accompanied him to the emergency room, or if she is present or absent during his hospital stay. The interview also tells us that the week of the stroke is full of special events that have all occurred during this time of year: the most active time each year in his work (in the hotel industry), the time when he does not have custody of his children, the time when he breaks with the "women of his life", the date of his mother's death, the date of his boss' death (whom he presents as a father figure) and the time of labyrinthine crisis (which goes very well with the character's discourse).

[19] We are in the presence of a classic case associating stroke with her own birthday here, celebrating her fiftieth birthday. Moreover, bordering on premeditation, this lady had predicted, the day before, the time of the stroke with the time of her birth (which had amazed her entourage). The lady also associates the number 50 with her parents' 50th wedding anniversary celebration, which she links to her mother's stroke one year before this anniversary.

[20] As soon as she knew she was pregnant, the young woman told

her parents, brother and sister-in-law. According to her, as soon as the couple heard the news, they set *to work* and, 9 months later, had a son. The young woman's stroke occurred at the parents' cottage a few days after the nephew's birth, when the whole family was gathered to celebrate the arrival of this new member. The young woman was accompanied by her husband and their three-month-old daughter, the brother, sister-in-law and newborn were at that time at rest (on parental leave). At the time the stroke symptoms appeared, the young woman was alone with her daughter in the living room, "her boyfriend had just left her", that is, according to her, he had just gone into the kitchen to join the rest of the family. Then a "real symptom of 15 minutes of reversed vision" occurred, with the participant seeing two scenes at the same time, the right eye seeing what the left eye was seeing and vice versa. The first consequence of a stroke will be that this woman will no longer be able to care for her daughter, that she will have to stop breastfeeding her, that she will become the centre of family attention again, always having someone to care for her, being dependent on a relative to prepare her meals and help her eat. She will then spend "a month of vacation" at the parents' cottage.

[21] This man tells us (with the help of his wife) that he has never been ill in his life, with the exception of two flu infections: the most recent one occurred a short time earlier, during the week between his birthday and his stroke (the first one seven years ago, when there was a major birth in his family). He adds jokingly that he was not allowed to be sick because he no longer had (due to administrative problems) a valid health insurance card. After taking steps to remedy this inconvenience, he finally receives his card a few days after his birthday and ironically declares to his wife: "Now I can be sick." To what the wife adds, with a laugh: "The next day he had a stroke."

[22] On the eve of the stroke, in the evening, the woman listened to her TV show, *Destinées, des affaires de famille*[32]. The next day was supposed to be the last day of work before the Christmas break, then "she would fall on vacation". According to her, the holiday season does not evoke anything special while, according to her mother (present at the interview), this period recalls the accidental death of her father's brother on December 24, at the age of 45 (he died suffocated during his sleep). Her daughter then promptly insists that, even if she remembers the death, it has nothing to do with her stroke (except that her stroke occurred when she herself was 45 years old). However, she associates stopping working with

---

32. *Note from translators:* Which could be translated *Destinies, family affairs.*

the darkest events of her life that happened eight years ago (since then, she has been taking antidepressants). These events concerned the father's secret illness, the dazzling pain he had to endure and the last days of his life. This lady has always been very close to her father and had to stop working to take care of him daily while he was terminally ill. The father's hidden illness seemed most abominable, to the point that the mother of this lady, when she became (too late) aware of his condition, could not have endured the horror of the thing, preferring that her daughter take care of it. The participant was the only witness to this descent into hell.

[23] This man (colourful, saucy, vulgar and uninhibited) tells us that very early in the morning (6:30 am), on day of his stroke (a few days after his birthday[33]), he called his best friend and asked him to come and see him that very day at 10:30 am, before he went to the Laurentians for the holiday season. However, he insists that he does not remember making this call. According to this friend, during this call, he told him that he would "not lock the door" and that he would only have to enter the apartment (as if there was something premeditated). Shortly before the appointment, the man took a shower, taking care not to close the bathroom door. At the agreed time, the friend entered the apartment, saw the body lying on the floor, naked in the bathroom, and called the paramedics. Friends, paramedics, landing neighbours would then all have entered the apartment to see the individual's "beautiful naked body", probably erect. The man ironicizes by pretending to be a former naked dancer, equipped with an oversized device.

[24] "Funny coincidence," said the young woman. Two children in this family, her and her brother. Her brother also has two children, who have the same age difference as between her and this brother. Two lives in parallel, in the same space, in the same work milieu, in the same environment, within the same social network, the same friends who all have the same life: the same number of children, in the same city, the same house, driving the same truck, holding the same profession, having the same debts, since adolescence in the same high school. In this stable life, in less than a month, two strokes, on the day of the meeting of two "ex", the two men "of her life", who are two exact copies of the young lady's brother, who have two new girlfriends, events that occurred on two Saturdays, the same scenario, a rupture that occurred twice during the holiday

---

33. It is interesting to note the individual's semantic exercise when questioned by the interviewer about possible birthdays or special events that may have occurred around mid-December. The latter replied, tacitly: "No, no, no, nothing special, I was born on December 15."

season (period especially overloaded with emotions in this family).

[25] The same day, shortly before the stroke, the woman said she had taken the time to advise her sister and a few friends not to forget to eat pancakes the next day, Friday the 13th, like at Candlemas. This practice of Candlemas (usually celebrated on February 2nd) ensures the person money and health for the rest of the year. On her part, the set-up for the next day's pancakes was already ready. The stroke itself occurred when the woman had just sat down, around 10 a.m., to watch her TV show[34]. She carefully recounts the activities surrounding stroke: sitting in front of the TV, going to the bathroom, going back to bed, staying in bed. She remembers all the details of this episode because her mother had experienced exactly the same scene on February 25th, 25 years earlier, on the day of her death, a sudden death while listening to *Le crime d'Ovide Plouffe*[35] at 10:00 p.m. She also associates her symptoms, arrhythmia and angina, with those who took her father away, still in February, 10 years earlier.

[26] This case history here highlights the ambivalence of stroke that precipitates the order of things, giving rise to what it had hindered. The young woman opened the interview by discussing the events surrounding her stroke; with her [new] lover, after making love, she was washing in the shower and suddenly felt a sharp headache, as if someone had hit her with a baseball bat. This stroke had for consequences to prevent the young woman from using contraception, and a possible pregnancy would become, according to her expression, "a calculated risk". Nevertheless, she became pregnant, a pregnancy that doctors feared, and had to inject herself into her belly at the beginning of her pregnancy. Consciously, she most likely wanted to get pregnant, but stroke showed that this decision was quite "risky". A second stroke, three months after delivery, will confirm the risk.

[27] The woman refers to a first stroke (which is not documented in the file) in the spring of 2011, five days of migraine when she thought she was pregnant. In the end, there will be no pregnancy. The second (?) stroke occurred when the woman was particularly hyperactive, as she had to complete the preparations for a cruise planned with her partner, a first attempt to leave alone, as a couple, to get away from their family responsi-

---

34. This Thursday's program focused on a new book by Marie Laberge, *Revenir de loin* (which can be translated *Come back from afar*), the story of a woman emerging from a coma who can no longer remember her life.

35. *Note from translators:* Which can be translated *The Crime of Ovide Plouffe,* who's suspected of killing his wife.

bilities. This cruise was to mark the couple's wedding anniversary. Stroke will prevent the event from happening. The woman is most aware of the ambivalence of the relationship with her partner and addresses the issue openly: she says she has seriously considered separation before the birth of their child; she talks about their sexual problem, childhood trauma and the partner's desire to have another child, which she does not want, and that she can no longer have because of the stroke. She describes her partner as a physically and psychologically frail being, a pink man, while she sees herself as a solid woman, never sick, "a mother in cement", surprised that the stroke "comes from her side and not from that of the spouse".

[28] Completely defensive, the individual begins the interview by saying he has memory problems, many gaps. During the first few minutes of the interview, there is an incalculable succession of "no, no, no, as usual, I don't remember, I have a blank, there's nothing, nothing special, really nothing really nothing, the routine". Nothing, no theme seemed to be associated with particular events that might have occurred around the few days before or after the stroke date. Nothing, until the spouse, who was present at the interview, clarifies that this date was associated with the subject's date of birth, her daughter's birthday, the participant's sister's birthday, and finally the participant's mother's stroke date (in fact, the events surrounding his stroke appear to mirror those of his mother's stroke). Stroke and its hospitalization will naturally cancel out the celebrations planned during this period.

[29] The man, awaiting a decision to obtain a disability pension following the stroke, seems to be convinced that the purpose of the interviewer's approach is to evaluate the services he receives to correct the financial lightness of his situation. He complains, explains and justifies the shortcomings of his care plan and lists in detail the many expenses required by his condition and disability. He also talks about the sums he has to pay to support his institutionalized and severely disabled son. While complaining about his lack of money, he explained that, during the month of the stroke, he had been informed of the increase in his rent. This stroke occurred while he was taking his annual vacation, during which time he usually takes the opportunity to visit his son. This year, stroke prevented these meetings.

[30] The stroke occurred after returning from a vacation in the South, when this man took his father's place to accompany his mother with a group of twenty-two members of the paternal family. This was the mother's first trip to the South (although the individual says he had already

taken her to Walt Disney[36]). This trip to the South had postponed a dental surgery that seemed meaningful to him (he did not want to start his trip under the effect of the drugs prescribed following his intervention): he had broken a tooth around the age of 30 (period that corresponds to the time of separation of the parental couple). The tooth was replaced, i.e., glued back together, on his return from the trip, the day after the father's birthday[37], five days before the stroke. This man lost his tooth twice during intubation procedures due to post-stroke hospitalization.

[31] During the stroke, the woman kept her grandson, her daughter's son, conceived *in vitro* (a second attempt at pregnancy, a few years later, had given no results). The lady recounts that her daughter had great difficulty *getting pregnant;* she describes her son-in-law as an old bachelor. The stroke therefore complicated her daughter's vacation, the regular babysitter had to come urgently to take care of the 8-year-old child, it should be noted that the woman has not seen her grandson since the stroke (the interview took place two months after the stroke). She recounts the details of the events surrounding the stroke when she was alone with her grandson at the child's home (note that it was Valentine's Day weekend). The day before, the lady was not in good shape, "having pain somewhere ", experiencing back pain. The grandson then took care of her, as during a game, taking her temperature, giving her massages, and giving her his father's syrup. That night, she slept with her grandson in his parents' bed. The next day, while her grandson was peeing, the lady urinated on the ground. The grandson told her to wash and lent her his father's boxers so she could change. It was a little later, while the lady was chatting with her daughter on the computer (Skype), that her daughter noticed the physiological manifestations of stroke (crooked mouth and eye problems). While the stroke took the woman away from her grandson, it did allow a connection with her own son; it was the latter who cared for her and stayed with her during the hospitalization (in any case, this son was always very close to the woman and had difficulty separating from her, which he finally did since his marriage, and since the birth of a little girl). The woman regrets that she did not have the energy to care for this 16-month-old granddaughter at the time of the interview. It should be noted that during the interview the lady intertwines the son's first name and the grandson's; she does not address the questions surrounding her family circle (no words about her mother, father, brother or sister) and she refuses to address the question

---

36.   Ironically, one might wonder if the subject is his mother's son, husband or father.
37.   The individual points out that his father had always been radically opposed to all forms of events that could mark his birthday.

of her religious devotion (why does a little candle constantly burn in her living room in front of a statue of the Virgin?).

[32] This man presents a rather peculiar character, obsessed with money issues; in fact, the interview was more like filing a large financial statement following an investigation by the revenue department. As soon as he discusses a character (spouse, father, mother, brothers, children, in-laws), he talks about his/her assets, properties, expenses, debts, investments, income, inheritance, professional status, etc. Money issues thus occupy all the remarks from the beginning to the end of the interview, the man listing in the smallest details his expenses, his debts, the costs he has had to bear and still has to bear. The stroke itself occurred on the weekend when the individual and his spouse were celebrating Valentine's Day, with a dinner and a show. The couple was absolutely determined to see this show. The man had purchased the tickets in mid-December (the date of his mother's birthday) to give to his spouse as a Christmas gift. Strangely, during the interview, the man was unable to remember the name of the artist he wanted to see on stage, he could only remember the title of this show *Man in Black* (After the interview, a search revealed that it was a *Tribute to Johnny Cash* [38].). It should be noted that stroke occurred a few days after his birthday (he associates the date of his stepfather's death with the passing of time, two days after his birthday, highlighting the importance of an inheritance issue that improves his poor financial situation). On the day of the show, the man had begun work at the residence of his brother-in-law (his spouse's brother), physically very demanding work, where he had to

---

38. We spontaneously named this case story Mr. *Johnny Cash*, this label representing better than any theoretical synthesis the essence of the issue of the scenario that is in question here. It is far from commonplace that the character featured in this show was forgotten, repressed by the participant, this signifier being indeed at the heart of this stroke. Note that the other cultural representations we have cited (movies, shows, public presentations, TV shows or series) that were consumed by some individuals at or shortly before the first manifestations of stroke symptoms – we think of a particular episode of the series Les Parent [in French, Parent is the surname of a family], or the series *Destinies*, the episode entitled *A Family Affair*, the program on Marie Laberge about her book *Come back from afar*, or the movie *The Crime of Ovide Plouffe* – were all very meaningful in successfully expressing, in a direct and succinct way, a vignette that was limited to the content of the case stories involved (it is not surprising that stroke occurs at this very moment). Freud placed this phenomenon on the side of an *Unheimlichkeit*, of a *disturbing strangeness* that violently shocks the subject at the moment when he/she "perceives", unconsciously, that what he/she is seeing expresses clearly and simply, without him/her being able to understand it, without him/her being able to knowingly name it, the essential part of what he/she lives in the depths of his/her intimacy. Unfortunately, as we see here, the content of this representation is often repressed, expelled from consciousness, and the individual remains unable to remember it.

redo, on his knees, four-legged, the concrete floor of a future washroom in the basement. The stroke had the inevitable effect of interrupting work on this site. In retirement, in need of income, he also talks about the work he had to do at the residence of his wealthy older brother, for a few dollars a week.

[33] The subject turns out to be a dyad in symbiosis (the man and his wife), two bodies, one mind, with the same pathologies, thyroid problems and stroke. The wife's mystical beliefs probably do not help the situation (a retired nurse who has premonitions and anticipates the future), so the man does not ask any questions and listens to his wife. For example, in month of the stroke, the participant's daughter (whom he associates with his sister) tells him that she is pregnant with her first baby. According to the wife, this pregnancy is associated with a risk of death, she had several feelings. The foetus will strangely die on the weekend following the stroke, on the wife's birthday. On stroke day, it was also the wife who noticed the first symptoms, exclaiming: "Hey, you're doing me a stroke." According to the wife, the sequence of events is as follows: her husband's sister's fatal cancer caused her death, her mother could not overcome this death and died, these two simultaneous deaths caused his hypertension which led to his stroke.

[34] The woman began the interview by presenting the events surrounding the stroke as the result of a shock associated with her mother's death two months earlier. This death would have caused her severe migraines that precipitated the stroke. The woman says she stayed with her mother for almost 40 years to care for her, but because she no longer had the health to care for her (because of the first symptoms of stroke), she had to make the decision to place her in an institution. This institutionalization had greatly disturbed the woman, to the point where, when she visited her (accompanied by her goddaughter), she saw her in her grave instead of in her bed. The stroke itself occurred on a Sunday evening when the woman was listening to TV tapes[39] with her goddaughter on her goddaughter 's birthday (she says she is very attached to her nephews and nieces, a compensation for not having had a child).

[35] Cacophonic interview: a problem of language, accent, communication, memory loss, imprecision, confusion, to which is added the discourse of the spouse who interferes in the remarks, censors, repeats, interprets, confronts. However, a knot of events seems to emerge clearly from the remarks: everything is played out in February, around the theme

---

39.   Unfortunately, it was impossible to know which programs were involved.

of marriage, between the day of his birthday and the end of February (anniversary of his last wedding), via the celebration of Valentine's Day. According to the medical chart, the stroke occurred on February 20 when he was convinced that it occurred on February 27. During this period, over the past three years, the individual recounts a few trips to the South to celebrate his marriage, the anniversary of his meeting with his new spouse and, subsequently, to celebrate the anniversary of that marriage. On stroke day, there is a vague reference to a dinner with friends (which will not take place) and a strange lady, the travel organizer, whom the man seems to know well (but whom the wife censors during the interview). The stroke allegedly occurred while he was alone with this lady. There is also mention of a first stroke the previous year, always during a trip to the South, at the same time of year, followed by memory loss (stroke not documented in the file).

[36] According to the lady, the thing is obvious: stroke is the direct consequence of her chemotherapy treatments for throat cancer. She associates this cancer with motherhood, as the cancer was triggered during her pregnancy. She also associates her symptoms with those of her mother: loss of voice, leftover tonsil debris and chronic sore throat. Permanently on antibiotics, her mother was unable to have children, but as soon as her tonsil debris was removed, she *became* pregnant. Unlike her mother's, the lady's cancer prevents her from having another child. She will have only one daughter whom she describes as her mirror, as herself very small with a very small voice. The participant recounts the recurrence of her cancer in 2012, 22 years (her daughter's age) after her first episode. She associates this period with her new spouse's stroke and her daughter's announcement to leave the family home in March of that year. We see how the cancer associated with the birth of her daughter and the recurrence of this cancer associated with the departure of this girl (stroke triggering event) are ambivalent. Cancer is the cause of her daughter's birth, but prevents her from having another child. In an equally ambivalent way, the lady, being funny, talks about her daughter as a cancer (astrological sign); she admits "it remains that she is my daughter" and talks about the 20% "chance" [she corrects herself], the "risk" of having a recurrence of her cancer.

[37] From the outset, the woman has defined herself as an addict for more than a decade, unfit for work, living on social welfare. She describes the events surrounding stroke and how, on that day, she was talking with her son and his friend after they had just smoked pot. She insists on specifying that this friend is not her son's girlfriend, but just a friend. "And then, all of a sudden, it happened. Other than that, I don't remember any-

thing else. Well, I remember telling my son that I wanted to go to bed, but when I got to my bed, I had a craving, so I asked him to take me to the bathroom, where he sat me on the bowl, then he kicked himself off the boat and went away. I fell down. I hit my head, I remember that, I hit my head on the terrazzo on the ground. It hurts."

[38] For this man, it is very clear that stroke is caused directly by overtraining in the gym, and a bad stretch that caused a dissection of the cerebral artery. During the previous month, on his 48th birthday, the man had made the decision to change his lifestyle to restore his health (he admits, towards the end of the interview, that it was a decision he bitterly regretted, and that he had started eating badly again, because "health is not good, it kills "). As for the events surrounding the stroke (although he insists that nothing special happened in the month it happened), the interview tells us that exactly one year before the stroke the man had decided to sell his business. So a year later, during the week of the stroke, the man felt ready to reinvest in a new business. He says the stroke has cost him a business opportunity (which we will never know). We also learn that the man owned several businesses for several years and that dishonest partners had often deceived him; he even lost a friend after 30 years of relationship because the latter had started stealing from him. At the time of the stroke, the man had therefore decided to embark on the adventure again with a new partner.

[39] The man recounts the events surrounding the stroke by explaining that on this Sunday in March, he was chatting on Facebook. He was alone at home, his spouse had left with her youngest daughter to visit her other daughter (the participant's two daughters-in-law). The man says [unfortunately] that he does not remember the content of the "chat" site he was visiting at the time (he does, however, remember meeting his new spouse accidently when "chatting" on Facebook). He describes the symptoms experienced during the stroke (phlebitis in the right leg and pulmonary embolism) and associates them with those of his father who died around the same date. He refers to March as *the* month of birthdays: in addition to the anniversary of his father's death, he celebrates his own birthday and that of his spouse (the day after his stroke). He adds that this year the stroke ensured that there was no celebration for his wife's birthday, stating, confidentially, that his relationship with his spouse is in danger.

In what way do these events become the circumstances of stroke?

2nd reduction, eidetic reduction

Based on the various events surrounding the onset of stroke, and based on the individual's discourse, here are (presented in alphabetical order of the name given to the case histories) the typically repressed meanings that manifest themselves and express themselves through the sense of the circumstances that determine stroke.

Thus (in most case histories[40]), the event that occurs vertically in front of the subject (1st reduction) actualizes, reminds, animates, resumes or revives horizontally an affective conflict that concerns the very circumstances that the consciousness cannot support or take charge of[41].

[*1*] The lady calls on a mystical heritage that makes the brilliant women of her clan mostly related to draft men who are quickly abandoned (which, according to her, will soon prove to be the case for her daughter). According to her, stroke is, still according to her, an act of protest against the fate cast on her clan; an act of radical rejection that should make her daughter understand and prevent her from being in contact with her son-in-law who is the roughest of men.

[*2*] The woman tells us that while she was kneeling in the sea and experiencing the first symptoms of her stroke, she was thinking about the fact that she was the same age as her father when he had his fatal heart attack. She also recounts that the setting reminded her of the journeys she made alone with her child, a child she considers most precious and which she almost tragically lost at the age of three.

[*3*] The participant describes himself as an alcoholic, an A.A. member for about thirty years, following the separation of his spouse. He says he is very involved in A.A.: the day after the stroke, he was supposed to host a major conference, but unfortunately, hospitalization prevented him

---

40. Either such circumstances simply do not exist in some cases, or the interview was unable to collaborate with the subject's defences to access them.

41. It should be noted that this second reduction cannot be understood as an entity independent of our first reduction; it is a complementary entity that clarifies, qualifies, circumscribes and emotionally explains a conflict that manifests the very meaning of stroke. It can thus be compared to a secondary elaboration of the analysis of the content of a dream. Unfortunately, as we were explaining, mainly for ethical reasons, we cannot present these two reductions one after the other without revealing information that may unveil the identity of the participants. The order of these two reductions has therefore been changed, the numbers here in italics not corresponding to those of the first reduction.

from carrying out his project (he will then ask his daughter to contact those in charge to announce the news and justify his absence). This 30-year-old girl is very present and important in his life. They have always lived together or in the same building. She has been living with her husband since the early 2000s, a couple that the individual has great difficulty accepting because, according to him, his son-in-law is putting his wife through an unbearable life[42]. A few days before the stroke, when celebrating his alcohol-free anniversary, he reportedly had a discussion with his son-in-law during which he was informed that he had just had a fight with his daughter and that they had made the decision to separate. This news affected the man enormously, who was then convinced that he was the main cause of the separation (this separation will eventually complicate his life, as the couple owns the building where they all three live). During the hospital stay following the stroke, the couple would have decided to resume living together and was still together at the time of the interview, three months later.

[4] On the morning of the stroke, this man said he had finally undertaken a major cleaning, the household of a lifetime, by attacking his basement, which has been storing his collections for 30 years: hundreds of objects related to the history of kitchen tools (which he called the objects of an anthropological heritage) and an impressive collection of images and representations of the mother goddess (among others the Venus of Willendorf, the first mother, "our mother to all"). The individual says he has worked all his life as a journalist, mainly in the area of women's issues. He retired in 1980, at the time of his mother's death. He said he was very close to this mother, named Maria, reproducing her lifestyle and taking up her interests. It is for this reason that he collected objects with such meticulousness (just like his mother, "it is certainly", according to him, "a genetic trait").

[5] The man presents himself as an individual who has experienced serious alcohol problems. He notes a series of associations linking two strokes to meaningful events in his life and talks about the ambivalence of the relationship with his ex-spouse, the ordeal of his marital life, his separation, an accident with his boss's car, the sale of his car and the suspension of his driver's licence (preventing him from working as a truck driver). In reviewing the events surrounding the last stroke, the participant

---

42. Let us note a comment from the subject stating that this son-in-law is a carbon copy of his brother, a brother with whom the individual has always been in deep rivalry and whom he has never been able to bear.

spontaneously associates it with the moment when he was "hugging his neighbour". He describes this neighbour, whom he never names, as "a gluer, an annoying", who has "a serious alcohol problem", stating that "it is her problem, not mine". He insists several times that this relationship is not meaningful to him, that he has not had another woman in his life since his ex-wife, that he is very well, not wanting to talk about this neighbour, preferring to change the subject, although, paradoxically, he sees her almost every day and that he does not worry about receiving help "since she is always there, next door".

[6] Mother of two children, this woman, whose mother tongue is French, explains how the effects of her stroke had the direct effect of preventing her from communicating in English with her family and friends (note that her spouse only speaks English). As for the children, she only speaks in English to her oldest (not her youngest), who has an English-speaking first name, the same first name as his father and grandfather. It should also be noted that during the interview she does not name him directly by his first name but speaks of "him" (eighteen times). Finally, it should be noted that the grandfather of the children (her husband's father) was a wonderful man who died of cancer five years ago, strangely enough on the same day she gave birth to her youngest child, two months before her stroke. However, she insists that this coincidence is not necessarily related to her stroke, although the time of year that corresponds to the arrival of this second child is symbolically overloaded with meaning.

[7] According to the participant, two heart ailments related to two family cases, five years apart, had announced this stroke. The first of these discomforts occurred when a niece (the daughter of his younger sister) was born, the second in the period between his birthday and stroke day. Unfortunately, serious memory problems and episodes of amnesia have hampered our understanding of the course of events. These include a serious disagreement with his father since his older sister became pregnant (in fact, he has not spoken to his father since that event) and a violent break-up with his brother since the stroke that killed his mother. At the time of the interview, the individual noted that his stroke had allowed him to initiate attempts to connect with his family.

[8] The participant began the interview by talking vaguely about the double stroke that took his mother away ten years ago, and the many nervous tics that date back to the time of his father's death, when the individual left his hometown and moved to Montreal. Then, he addresses the trauma of his life: the birth of his son with severe cerebral palsy. He describes this son as a monster, an inhuman beast, a violent creature, against nature,

indomitable, tossed from one institution to another, from one foster family to another, abused and beaten. The day of the stroke should correspond to the beginning of the annual period during which the man usually visited his son. That year, the visit will not take place.

[9] This lady was repulsive of everything to do with relationships. The meaning she gives to her stroke is naturally linked to this repulsion. However, she agreed to talk about her ex-spouse, the shock of the separation when this spouse decided to leave her on December 24 to go with his secretary ("a slap in the face") and the deep depression that followed the event. She also tells us about her best friend from childhood, who had the same first name as her, a good travel friend who suffered the same fate as her about the adventure she had with her husband. She describes her great sorrow when this friend died of cancer after great suffering. Finally, let us note the importance of the theme of massage (and personal care) that recurs throughout the interview. She tells how a man bought her ex-husband's house, this man was a masseur, "my God he was giving good massages". The lady then talked about it with her friends and quickly built him up a large clientele. She remembers with emotion the massages of this man and this period of her life (which she links with the presence of her best friend).

[10] The individual's main memories all come back to 10 years ago (fall 2001) at the defining moment of his life when he retires, quits smoking, stops drinking and splits up with his wife. It should be noted that 10 years to the day before the stroke occurred, it was September 11, 2001, the fateful day of the attacks in New York City recalled by all the media in September 2011 (most likely acting as a memory trigger).

[11] The participant presents a classic family history worthy of the greatest oedipal scenarios. "The clan", as he calls it, does not seem to be affected by the prohibition laws that usually separate symbolic and generational ties. The eldest of the grandchildren of his generation, the man is the same age as his mother's cousins, whom he considers to be his own cousins. He is also the same age as his mother's younger brothers, he talks about his uncles like his friends, like his brothers; the latter call him "their second-bed brother". Finally, he considers his maternal grandmother as his cousin's second mother. This generational ambiguity, even *incestuous*, goes beyond the limits of his own clan: the mother's ex-sister-in-law happened to be his cousin and his brother is in a relationship with the father's ex-girlfriend. His parents are separated, the individual claims to be responsible for this separation, it is he who forced his father to leave his mother. He describes his father as a "philanderer alcoholic", he says that he would

have other children in another city, naturally with other women. He adds that he has cut off ties with him, that he does not need him in his life, that this story is currently going on six feet above his head and that he is now taking on the role of father, assuming the responsibilities of the father. He added that the whole family on the mother's side was very happy with the separation and that, in the end, "he had done a good deed". Stroke will necessarily be related to this type of family scenario and separation.

[*12*] The woman spontaneously associates her stroke with migraines she has been experiencing since she was 14 years old, when she had her first period. However, she links the intensity of her last migraines leading to stroke to a period of deep depression that occurred 15 years ago, when she was due to marry. Her state of health meant that she had to postpone the wedding until the following year. She adds that, during the preparations for this wedding, she discovered a lump on her breast that turned out to be a cancerous tumour. After the operation to remove this tumour and several chemo and radiotherapy treatments, a precancerous calcification of the breast led to a partial mastectomy. An apparently innocuous detail, it should be noted that the lady points out that the first symptoms of stroke appeared when she was "decalcifying" her snow boots (i.e., cleaning traces of calcium) and that she associates the episode of gallstones and digestive hemorrhages with the symptoms (and her genetic background) of her dead mother.

[*13*] The stroke occurred during the Christmas holiday break, when the young lady met her ex-boyfriend with her new pregnant girlfriend. She says she turned white as a dead woman, started shaking and having convulsions. This ex-boyfriend would be a true copy, in all respects, of his father. This holiday season seems most meaningful to her, recognizing that the period may be associated with an old stress experienced by her father and admitting that "especially in her family the holiday season is overloaded with emotion". The image of the father returns to the heart of the interview when the young woman associates her age at the time of the stroke (25 years) with the age of the father who, at 25 years of age, "leaves" his mother and the family home and meets a new woman who will become his spouse (the subject's mother). In fact, the paternal grandmother would have thrown her son out because he had huge alcohol problems ("my father, at 25, he would come home to my grandmother dead drunk every night"). She adds that it was during the holiday season that the father, several years later, made the decision to stop drinking. Finally, it should be noted that this father's character seems quite particular; according to the young lady, he had, still according to her, several extramarital

relationships and several illegitimate children.

[*14*] A clan of women: the subject, her mother and daughter. Her mother speaks, the subject listens, submissive and nodding. No trace of a man in 20 years. Either they have disappeared or died (subject's spouse, paternal uncle or mother's brother-in-law). Ironically, the subject's father was born with a genital malformation and would have only a small piece of penis. How did this penis manage to procreate? This parental couple did not seem to be heading in the right direction (any more than the other couples who make up this women's clan). As the subject's mother says: "This penis malformation is the worst case, I wouldn't wish it on my best, on my, on my worst enemy." As this slip of the tongue indicates, the couple's ambivalence was obvious. Was the couple sterile? "I was hard to get pregnant; we don't know why. We never did any tests on it, but I was due to have a child." After nine years of marriage (and attempts), their only child will be born, premature, after seven months of pregnancy, but also with a birth defect: a heart murmur and a three-inch hole in the heart. Over time, "the hole in the heart disappears, but the heart murmur gets worse". Still according to the mother, she was convinced that the subject's stroke was "a kind of fatality due to her birth; the heart murmur turned into a clot that went up to her brain[43]".

[*15*] This case story features another case of a women's clan. The lady, a retired professional, lives in her own little world, surrounded by her sister and a few friends. There has been no man in her life for several years and she says she hates children. She is talking about another sister, with whom she has severed ties and has had no contact since her father's death, a matter of money and inheritance manipulation. She also talks about a good friend, "like a sister", who died of cancer last March. The lady sees the stroke (which also occurred in March) as a memorial ceremony, in memory of the father, who died of a heart attack, always and again in March, almost 10 years ago. According to her, stroke is there to show which of the two rival sisters is closest to the father and naturally deserves his legacy.

[*16*] Still under the theme of fratricidal rivalry, this elder, constantly supplanted by his younger brother, had agreed (before the stroke) to participate in a family celebration lasting a few days (at his parents' estate) to mark the birth of a first nephew in the family (i.e., his rival brother's son). The stroke occurred shortly before this celebration, so for one of the first

---

43. Let us highlight here the power to prescribe and the impact, in the discourse of those around us, of an organization of genetic predispositions.

times in his life, it was the participant who passed as the focus of the family's attention, relegating his brother, wife and nephew to the background. In fact, the individual does not recall seeing the young infant during his stay.

[*17*] Another case of fratricidal rivalry this time involves the younger brother who, according to his expression, spent his life "on his knees" in front of his older brothers (often serving them as cheap labour for thankless tasks). When the first symptoms of stroke broke out, he was precisely "four-legged" in his brother-in-law's basement digging a hole that would eventually serve as a site for a future toilet.

[*18*] To this young lady's great disappointment, the hospitalization following the stroke will prevent her from being present at the birthday celebration (prepared long ago) celebrating her daughter's 18th birthday. The interview tells us that this girl is an adopted child. From the beginning of her new cohabitation, this baby turned out to be a problem child, her babysitter was telling incredible things about her, the spouse had to stop working to take care of her. A medical assessment, when the girl was 2 years old, confirmed a diagnosis of autism. It should be noted that the child was named Marguerite[44] to recall the memory of the subject's sister, who tragically died at the age of 18 from a road accident at the time of adoption.

[*19*] This man, with a strong psychiatric background, is experienced with introspection and guided interviews. He was surprised by the freedom of association granted him by the phenoanalytical interview and agreed to submit to it without opposition. This open-mindedness allows him, from the beginning of the interview, to make connections that force him to reconsider the story he normally repeated to anyone who wants to hear it. Thus, he quickly realized that the episodes of confusion he mechanically referred to in 2002 had in fact begun in September 2001 and that they were associated with the tragic events of September 11. We then understand differently the dynamics that manifested the stroke at the time of the 10th anniversary of this tragedy (September 2011). Similarly, by reviewing the sequence of events, he spontaneously notes that he was, in September 2001, the same age as his mother at the time of her death.

[*20*] The woman recounts that stroke day was "a strange date" that commemorated the day when her police husband – about ten years ago, shortly before she left – reportedly threatened her with death with his gun (his police colleagues would then have intervened to control him). She

---

44. Analogous first name.

says today that she is far from these disturbing events in her emotional life and is happy to be accompanied by a new spouse who, strangely enough, is also a police officer and, according to several clues given by the woman, just as violent as her ex-spouse.

[21] The participant, claustrophobic, associates the position in which he felt paralyzed the night he experienced stroke symptoms with the memory of being trapped overnight in his baby bed at age two in a hallway while his mother was in her room caring for the younger brother shortly after his birth. It is interesting to note that the date of the accidental death of this brother, who over time had become his rival, is associated by the individual with that of stroke.

[22] The events surrounding the stroke evoked the possibility of conflict in this woman's marital life. The ambivalence of the relationship with the spouse seemed obvious. Sleeping in a separate room seemed to satisfy the lady, because she was snoring and her partner could hardly stand her presence at night. This spouse did not seem interested in family life, he was absent during the woman's delivery and quickly went on a trip after the delivery. According to the lady, this man was having difficulty managing his affective and sexual life; she hoped that stroke could bring the couple together, but in vain. She associates her husband with her father, a "philanderer" who uses all pretexts to escape the marital home. To overcome this uncomfortable situation, the woman calls herself a *workaholic* and talks about a meaningful relationship with a colleague (whom she calls "her boyfriend" during the interview), with whom she had spent the evening the night before the stroke. The importance of the woman's professional career seems undeniable, she lives only for her work and occupies functions usually reserved for men (it should be noted that her father exercised the same profession).

[23] This man's stroke occurred on his spouse's birthday and naturally prevented celebrations to mark the occasion. When asked about his relationship with his spouse, the individual describes this "new" spouse as a woman with a lot of character who did not have it easy, her ex-husband having committed suicide (hanged in the family home, she found him). He points out that he had known this woman for a few years, an ex-in-law relationship. He says "that he hit a good woman" and insists that he does not experience more conflicts than other couples, although it is not always easy. However, he recounts (which he considers regrettable) that he moved to this new spouse's home, in a new region, leaving behind his mother, his three daughters and his ex-spouse in his hometown.

[*24*] The stroke was directly related to the theme of this woman's maternity, it occurred while she thought she was pregnant. In her family, issues related to pregnancy and childbirth have always been ambiguous, constantly associated with complications (caesarean section, cancer, radiation therapy during pregnancy, abortion, etc.). Both her own birth (at the place and time of the grandmother's death) and her mother's other pregnancies were difficult. Despite this, this family "defect" suits the lady, because "it questions the legitimacy of her mother as a mother". The woman insists that if, like her mother, she had a stroke, hers showed that she had a heart while her mother's showed that she did not.

[*25*] Three years ago, in March, "crooked eye" vision problems forced the man to abandon his professional activities. At the same time, his mother agreed "under threat and abuse" to sign a power of attorney to his brother-in-law, "a crooked character, an unscrupulous bandit with a tie", naming him the sole inheritor of her property. According to the participant, his mother would only survive a few months in this constraining situation and would die in the same year. According to him, it was this conflictual atmosphere that led him to his stroke.

[*26*] This lady recounts, a notable fact, that at the time of the stroke she had to go to court to settle a dispute over her mother's estate. Her stroke prevented the hearings from being held, which were postponed to a later date (not yet determined at the time of the interview). This fact is far from insignificant when we make an after-the-fact connection with information obtained at the beginning of the interview regarding the circumstances surrounding the death of this woman's father. We had learned that this father had died 10 years earlier, as a result of a general deterioration in his health caused by a road accident that occurred while he was going to court to testify at hearings concerning a dispute over a question of money left as an inheritance to be shared between his family members. This association of facts was not identified during the interview, so we do not believe that the woman was conscious of it.

[*27*] First, let's note that this lady describes herself as a depressive schizophrenic. She recounts the stroke scene and that plunges her back into a vividly-remembered scenario that she associates with the living conditions she was living twelve years earlier, a time that seemed traumatic when she seriously started using drugs. At that time, she was living with a group of young people, including her eldest daughter and her friends. She would then have had a passionate relationship with her daughter's boyfriend, who was only 18 when she was more than 40. This adventure gave rise to a story as unimaginable as it was incredible, which would

end in a very bad outcome and would involve the intervention staff of the Youth Protection Directorate (YPD), street gang members, police arrests and court charges.

[*28*] This case history introduces ambivalent circumstances that will set the stage for a theme that we will have to develop. This is another apparently innocuous detail, but one that deserves special attention. This man's stroke occurred in the evening, when his spouse is systematically absent every week. The man knew, having noticed it several times, that at that time his neurologist neighbour was usually at home. As soon as the first signs of stroke appeared, the man contacted his neighbour who intervened urgently and personally accompanied him in the admission process and throughout his hospital stay (this neighbour was identified by the participant as "his relative" for the purposes of the medical file). This indirect, even ambivalent way of relating to another person is very unusual. This singularity effect seems to be a trait of character in this individual, which explains the feeling of ambiguity that bound him to his father until he saw in his father's death "the most beautiful thing I have ever contemplated during the whole of my life".

[*29*] An ambiguous, ambivalent, recalcitrant, even gruff participant who does not open up to the interview, making extensive use of saying "nothing" (more than thirty times during the interview), "no, nothing special" (as if he had things to hide). While he registers, when administering the socio-demographic questionnaires, as a single person living alone, he describes his activities of daily life using the pronoun "we"; while he never stops talking about his lifelong friend and alter ego, he promptly denies being or having been in relationship with the latter (yet it is obvious that he assumes his homosexuality and has nothing to hide about his sexual orientation). He associates the date of the stroke with a sister's and brother's birthday weekend, stating that "birthdays don't bother me," insisting that these birthdays are of no interest to him, except to give him the opportunity to think about his mother who, on that day, brought him into the world (the interviewer points out that a picture taken when the mother was a young girl stands in the centre of the main room of his home, while we find no trace or picture of a father or a male character). He says that the weekend before the stroke, he went to the movies as usual with his alter ego, that it was the Oscar weekend, but he is (unfortunately) unable to remember the movie they saw then. On the other hand, this interview is remarkable for showing us a new example of the symbolic importance of numbers[45]

---

45.   It should be noted that this individual is a mathematician.

that move on both temporal axes in a vertical and horizontal dimension, presenting the signifiers "forty", "twenty" and "twelve" in the same space, expressing both a decisive age and an equally decisive elapsed time (thus, "the age of 40 years" is condensed with "40 years ago"). We also hear the participant say that he has known his alter ego since the age of 12, that they both left their hometowns to come and live in Montreal in 1972. He talks about his 40-year depression, a period of shock of a strong existential crisis which he felt in his "forties", a time when he cut off ties with his brother with whom he had the best affinities and whom he had not seen for 20 years; he adds that he quit smoking "at the very age of 40, 20 years ago, that he had been living happily in Montreal for 40 years", etc. Finally, it should be noted that the individual claims to have no memory of his father or his death, which allegedly occurred on May 12. Let us conclude by saying that the stroke occurred in 2012 and that, when he was hospitalized, the delusional man was convinced that he was alive and well in 1972, being unable to remember the name of the institution in which he was living at the time, namely "Notre-Dame"[46].

[30] Another painful interview to follow. The confused character, nearly 70 years old, erratic, is difficult to understand with statements that similarly confuse the two temporal axes, whereas "when I was 18" condenses with "18 years ago", i.e., a speech intertwining memories of 1962 with others of 1994. The participant refers to heart conditions that are not documented in the file. An immigrant in Quebec at the age of 18, he then told us about a heart failure in front of a woman school principal; he also told us about another heart condition 18 years ago, while attending a neighbour's wedding when he was dancing with a man, South American. With regard to the current stroke, the one of particular interest to us, it should be noted that it also occurred in the presence of a female figure of authority in a South American context. Let us conclude by saying that this man went into exile to escape the control of his father and brothers (they, the individual himself and other family members all work in the same artistic profession). We note a definite ambivalence towards them on his part and we underline the same ambivalence in this man's mind about a struggle with homosexual ideas that he is trying to repress.

[During the study, we met a few individuals – mostly men – who were in a virile struggle against the existence of homosexual components. In psychopathology, this form of struggle is one of the most pernicious manifestations of the defences of the psychic system. In 1910, Freud made

---

46. Notre Dame could be translated in English as Our Lady.

this struggle against a homosexual component the trigger for a jealousy delirium that would prove to be a border between ordinary neurotic repression and devastating psychotic defences. Here is a sequence of case stories related to damage caused by demonstrations of this struggle.]

[*31*] This man, in a profound struggle against his homosexual components, explains that he could not bear the fact of "appearing as a homosexual". When he was living in a cohabitation with a woman, he said he was protected against this kind of offence. However, nearly 25 years ago, his wife decided to leave him. Collapsed, the individual was struck by a first heart attack. He says that this kind of heart disease "which had gotten the better of his father" allowed him to say: "I am just like my father, a philanderer who is not a homosexual." He also recounts that, "without his wife, having no children, he now ran the risk of looking as a homosexual". At the time, he had therefore immediately taken steps "to find a new spouse", which did not take long. Everything was going well in his life until this new spouse had her turn to leave him after 25 years of living together. The day she officially left the marital home, he contacted her and left her the following message: "You have to come back, I'm waiting for the paramedics, I had a stroke."

[*32*] Another man – a member of the Armed Forces and struggling with this virile protest against the existence of a homosexual component – recounts that the first symptoms of his stroke appeared as he undressed in the locker room before going to the communal showers. He also said that he noticed that day in the shower that his new chief adjutant, his primary hierarchical supervisor, "didn't have much leadership". The interview with this individual, despite his glacial appearance as a deadpan, was full of these kinds of expressions on the borderline between a slip of the tongue and a sauciness; it was impossible to know whether these expressions were voluntary or betrayed a deep existential unease. Living permanently with a group of men, far and away from "the slander and gossip of women's shrew", he also says he is safe from homosexuals, "because no faggot would be tolerated in the group". The older man tells of living with his mother all along, but sometimes refers to "the woman and her child". When asked about this by the perplexed interviewer, we learn that he is married, has a wife and at least one child, but is not interested in addressing the issue. The interview constantly returns to the character of the mother who is omnipresent, seeming to be the only meaningful person around him, with the exception of his one and only friend, José (whose name is written without "e" – Josée would be the feminine spelling – and he insists on this detail several times), whom the individual considers as

a brother, with whom he "slept all his childhood". Finally, he says he is not sure, despite doctors' diagnoses, that his vascular incident is a stroke because "his 75-year-old mother never had one".

[*33*] This manly participant, who is obviously a fierce homophobe, denies and ridicules his feminine side and all forms of weakness that would turn out to be an emotional burden. This struggle against this feminine side has cost him the price of a deep depression. However, his attending physician, a neighbour and childhood friend, comforted him by assuring him that the type of depression that had struck him had no psychological cause or impact and turned out to be a purely physiological phenomenon, in the order of a chemical disorder. Strange coincidence, during the interview, every time the individual wants to talk about "this great boyfriend", his tongue forks and pushes him to say: "my beautiful great boyfriend" or "he's a handsome doctor" instead of saying "a great doctor" (he blushes every time and gets over it). Equally strangely, when this doctor explained the biological reasons for his depression, he compared it to a stroke or used stroke as an example (well before the participant's stroke). It seems that the individual has fully understood the message. During this stroke, it was his neighbour doctor who intervened on the front line and took special care of him throughout his hospitalization and rehabilitation.

[This type of event leads us to see stroke as an act of action[47] that displays one or more components that are consciously and usually inhibited. Let us think, under the same theme, of the case history [23] of our 1st reduction which evokes stroke as a premeditated "act" allowing the individual to expose his homosexual component which is usually repressed manfully by the me-conscious.]

[*34*] Still on the subject of repressed or ambiguous homosexual demonstrations, the story of a woman who tells how the first symptoms of stroke occurred at the end of a martial arts session when she greeted her training partner (girlfriend and co-worker). She would then suddenly feel a numbness in her tongue. It is this girlfriend, in front of her, who would have noticed the complete asymmetry of her face. She adds that this stroke occurred on her wedding anniversary. This married woman, mother of a child, then discusses the ambivalence of her marital situation, stating that it is an anecdote about a homosexual relationship in her spouse's family that triggered an interest in him, which would quickly turn into a love at first sight. In discussing this theme, she explained that her father's name

---

47. Let us recall the case histories [16] or[19] in the previous section to convince us of this.

was Michel Girouard[48], highlighting the difficulties that this homonymous man could have brought during his lifetime (it should be noted that in Québec Michel Girouard's name is mainly associated with the cause and rights of homosexuals). However, she would like to maintain this bond and name her son "Girouard" so that the child does not lose this symbolic trace by bearing the name of his biological father, that is, the family name of her spouse. Finally, let us note that this lady lives in a world composed essentially of women: being the only one to have children in her family (including that of her spouse), she talks about her sister who has no boyfriend, her aunt who lives alone, her main girlfriends, her boss and says she is surrounded by a team of health workers, strictly composed of women (doctor, neurologist, psychotherapist, etc.).

[Let us finish this section by addressing a theme parallel to the one we are currently focusing on, which concerns, using similar logic, the existence of a perverse component that hinders the individual's balance.]

[*35*] This is a man who explains how deeply his life has been disrupted by the simple encounter with a character he absolutely cannot see or support. According to him (and obviously), stroke is directly related to the presence of this repulsive character. It should be noted that this character's name is Léopold Dion[49] and that this name turns out to be the homonym of another character who sordidly marked the history of Québec at the time and in the region where the participant lived during his childhood. Léopold Dion is a criminal and sex offender, pedophile and serial killer who, in the 1960s, was nicknamed "the monster of Pont-Rouge". It is interesting to note how intensely paedophile stories have always disturbed this individual's peace of mind and the number of episodes of the kind he has had to deal with over the course of his life.

---

48. Name naturally analogous.
49. Again, this is an analog name.

ANALYSIS OF SECONDARY THEMES

This is a summary of the information collected during the study regarding: 1) the reasons or causes (which we identify as *Gegenstände*) given by participants to justify their stroke; 2) *substrates* or the genetic (hereditary) luggage always given by the same participants to answer medical questionnaires that are constantly sent to them during their hospitalization; and 3) the physical locations where the first stroke symptoms appeared. This is a summary presentation because these three themes were not systematically documented during the interview; they were not part of the content to be covered in the interview guide. We want to present them because, after having found their relevance in the analysis of verbatim, we believe that they can provide an interesting perspective for a secondary analysis.

Finally, we present a list of the consequences directly mentioned by participants as having been caused by their stroke. Unlike the other three, this theme was covered by the theoretical rationale of the interview guide and was included in the interviewer's notebook.

Gegenstände

In our second part we wrote that we must start from the principle of putting in brackets (*épochè*) all forms of judgments or beliefs that make the phenomenon studied (in this case stroke) an extra-mental phenomenon (*Gegenstand*), i.e., existing in itself, as well as outside a meaningful or intentional link. We therefore hear the discourse of the stroke subject that explains to anyone who wants to hear it the reasons or causes that have caused, or strongly influenced, the occurrence of this stroke, in the sense of a *Gegenstand*, i.e., a private rationale used by the individual to reassure him/herself and give external meaning to his/her stroke (making his/her stroke an extra-mental phenomenon).

Thus, here are, in alphabetical order, the reasons or causes given by participants to give private meaning to their stroke.

List of *Gegenstände*

• A blow of fate	• Heat wave
• Act of God	• Household of a lifetime
• Bad luck	• Hugging her neighbour
• Biological fatality (2)	• Hyperactivity due to travel arrangements
• Can finally afford to be sick	• Hypertension
• Congenital complications	• Legacies of the mother
• Consequence of chemotherapy	• Little madness of the head
• Consequence of good lifestyle habits	• Mother's genome
• Consequence of sedentary life	• Mystical coincidence
• Diabetes	• Overtraining at the gym
• Diabetes, hypercholesterolemia	• Physical effort (layout)
• Drug's side effect	• Physical exhaustion
• Eating breakfast	• Physical phenomenon
• Emotional shock following a meeting	• Predestination
• Excess alcohol	• Professional exhaustion
• Fatal date	• Shock following the mother's death
• Fatigue	• Stress associated with family conflicts
• Following a training accident	vStress at work
• Generational conflict (daughter and son-in-law)	• Tracing the signs of a neighbour's stroke
• Genetically programmed	• Trauma anniversary

Substrates

It should be noted, as mentioned above, that the substrate of the stroke experience is and remains the subject's body in its reality (and in its bio-genetic heritage). The meeting of the vertical and horizontal axes is thus merged into the real body of an individual. Stroke is a real phenomenon; it is a manifestation in reality, the body of the individual suffers from it in its entirety, in his/her daily life, in his/her physical and psychological reality, as well as in his/her relationship with others. However, it should be noted that even if stroke is a real phenomenon, it does not make real the reason for stroke, its cause or trigger.

The following is an alphabetical list of hereditary medical reasons that participants use to justify (or strongly influence) the occurrence of their stroke.

List of genetic substrates

• Alcoholism (7)	• Father's heart disease (4)
• Arrhythmia	• Genetic determination
• Blood too thick (genetic)	• Heart disease (2)
• Chronic pain	• Infertility (5)
• Claustrophobia	• Inheritance of cardiac symptoms from the father
• Deadly motherhood	• Maternity cancer
• Deafness or balance problem	• Mother's breast cancer (2)
• Death on birthday dates (family and in-laws)	• Mother's cancer (3)
• Depression (3)	• Mother's heart disease (2)
• Diabetes	• Mother's heart disease and 2 strokes
• Drug addiction (4)	• Mother's heart disease and stroke
• Family heart disease	• Nervous ticks since the father's death
• Father's and mother's heart disease	• Psychosis (2)
• Father's alcoholism (2)	• Stroke subject somatise mimicry mother's stroke
• Father's Alzheimer's (not remembering)	• Sudden death of the mother of the family (cardiac arrest)
• Father's cancer (2)	• Vision problems

Locations

Here is a list, always in alphabetical order, of the physical locations where the first symptoms of stroke occurred.

List of locations

• Boat	• Lakefront
• Campsite	• On the way to a judicial appearance
• Country house (4)	• On the way to physiotherapy
• Gym (2)	• On the way to the gym
• Home (15)	• On the way to work
• Home (bathroom)	• Restaurant with son
• Home (shower) (2)	• Shopping centre
• Home (toilet or room)	• Sports room
• Home (toilets) (3)	• Travelling in the South
• Hospital	• Work (4)

Incidentally, let us note, the number of strokes for which the first symptoms are related to the bathroom (toilet) or have occurred in this room. In our society, the "bathroom", also called the "toilet" or "toilet room", is a very special place; it is the place of an intimacy reserved for the individual, no matter where he/she is (at home, at another person's home or in a public place). In this place (and almost exclusively in this place), the individual can have access to a private, locked, usually well-lit space in front of a mirror, where he/she can undress, meet basic needs, wash or even take drugs in privacy and without others' knowledge. This den of intimacy is far from trivial and can well serve as a place to express the most secret manifestations, coming from the deepest part of the human soul.

Effects (consequences) of stroke: benefits and disadvantages, advantages and impediments

Before the study began, we had planned to present the effects (or consequences) of stroke as perceived by participants and group them under two headings: 1) benefits and advantages and 2) impediments and disadvantages. We quickly realized that this task was just as impossible to determine as it was to classify; some consequences that, according to common sense, gave every reason to believe that they seemed most appropriate, if not positive, were perceived, according to participants, as extremely negative or unfortunate[50]. Thus, consequences such as "not having another child" or "not sleeping with a spouse" were expressed as favourable, while a "closer relationship with the spouse" was conflictive.

In the same way, very often, a cancelled event or opportunity, which could be or seem most pleasant, was probably perceived by the individual as a traumatic, terrorizing event, at the very least overloaded with ambivalent affects for the consciousness. How do we decide between all this?

We have simply decided to use the term "consequences" and leave the question of benefit or advantage, disadvantage or impediment open.

---

50. The frankness of these perceptions and the honesty of the discourse that recounts them are once again made possible only through the form of the interview guide, which, by simply giving a voice to stroke, allows transparency that is as rare as it is impossible to refuse. It seems that, for the majority of participants, there can be no question of not taking advantage of such a situation or of refusing such an opportunity for sincerity, which can only be the most beneficial, salutary and unique so that the word can approach recognition.

List of consequences

• Abandonment of professional activities	• Cancellation of dinner with friend (confidante)
• Absence of children	• Cancellation of dinner with friends
• Allowance, pension for disabled son	• Cancellation of dinner with sister-in-law
• Attention/mother's care	• Cancellation of joint anniversary dinner
• Attention/son's care	• Cancellation of judicial appointment
• Avoid A.A. convention	• Cancellation of meals with children in conflict
• Avoid being on vacation	• Cancellation of psychiatric appointment
• Avoid finding son who committed suicide	• Cancellation of restaurant (sister's birthday)
• Avoid labour disputes	• Cancellation of son's move
• Avoid the sworn enemy	• Cancellation of stay with uncles
• Avoid visiting brother	• Cancellation of the annual country house meeting during the holidays
• Become a centre of attention again	• Cancellation of wedding anniversary celebrations
• Being seen naked by a friend	• Cancels a friend's (ambivalent) flight adventure
• Being similar as a spouse	• Cruise cancellation (wedding anniversary)
• Breakdown of daughter's couple	• Disability pension
• Bring closer daughter	• Distancing of grandchildren
• Bring closer daughter's couple	• Distancing of the brother
• Bring closer friend's neurologist	• Do not invest money in the company
• Bring closer friend's physician	• Do not visit your son
• Bring closer mother	• Excluded from the sports team
• Bring closer nephew	• Forgetting nightmares
• Bring closer son (2)	• Getting help at home
• Bring closer the spouse	• Insurance bonus (work)
• Can help daughter	• Interrupt bathroom work
• Can no longer breastfeed	• Keep children away from the house
• Cancel daughter's birthday celebration	• Leave from work
• Cancellation of a romantic cruise	• Loss of speech
• Cancellation of annual trip to the South	• Money to take care of the son
• Cancellation of birthday celebrations	• Never to see your grandson again
• Cancellation of birthday meal	• No longer see (reverse vision)
• Cancellation of celebrations (several birthdays)	• No more hearing
• Cancellation of dental surgery	

• No more pregnancies	• Presence of an ambivalent friend
• No more responding to requests from brothers and brothers-in-law	• Preventing spouse from leaving
• No more seeing (spouse in the bath)	• Rejection of the son's coming-out
• No more sleeping with spouse	• Retirement
• No more taking care of children	• Sleeping with her daughter (need for comfort)
• No more taking care of your mother	• Supersede brother
• Not being alone anymore	• Suspension of driving licence
• Not having another child (2)	• Taking charge of own health
• Not to be contacted by spouse	• Travel cancellation (and indebtedness)
• Pension and social assistance	• Trip cancellation (2)
• Pensions (2)	• Unable to work (6)
• Permanent social assistance (2)	• Vision problem
• Postpone wedding	• Vision problems

PART 5

CONCLUSION

FOR A HOLISTIC PREVENTION OF STROKE

The results of this work show that the occurrence of stroke *on that day* is not exclusively a coincidence. This makes it important to recognize that each person is unique and that, despite genetic predispositions or healthy or unhealthy lifestyles, stroke symptoms, typically triggered by stress, manifest themselves in a complex but not trivial way. The current trend in our health care system is precisely to adopt a more client-centred approach, one that recognizes the need to take into account the patient experience. This trend is reflected, among other things, in the promotion of concepts such as health literacy, where the importance of communication being at a level that is understandable to all parties, or patient-partner, where the patient is enabled to make informed choices in relation to his/her life journey.

The phenomenological interview is a method that goes in this direction. It offers a space in which the person (the patient) can express self, starting from his/her symptoms, on what has meaning in his/her life (the signifiers), at this moment in his/her journey. These signifiers inform both the patient and health professionals about the affective, social and symbolic environment that influences the individual's health status. Thus, this approach is intended to be complementary to the traditional biomedical approach. It should be noted that, during a phenomenological interview, all subjects are allowed, even those (and probably especially those) that may surprise and seem to have no direct connection with health status. By giving the person the opportunity to express themselves freely, the themes addressed can only be related, important, relevant and meaningful. Consequently, one of the expected purposes of secondary prevention would be to allow the person to express self freely, to offer a space for speech where all topics of discussion are allowed and where necessarily the signifiers related to a node contributing to the health situation will be addressed. The individual stressors of each person can thus be detected and considered during secondary prevention. This work of recognizing or identifying the individual's own stressors is made possible by the layout of the phenomenological interview. It should be noted that an interview of less than one hour is sufficient for an interviewer with adequate training to identify these stressors, which makes this type of approach quite feasible in a clinical context.

Some themes or topics of discussion were found to be common, i.e., shared by several participants. As a result, it may be tempting to create a checklist with pre-established questions to ask all people who have had a stroke. However, this would be a mistake since the expressed ambivalence or over-investment in the relationship was, in the majority of cases, unknowingly unrecognized. Indeed, the interviewer had to be on the lookout for defence mechanisms to defuse them where possible, demonstrate openness and be attentive to the signifiers expressed by simply repeating them, while asking for symbolic details such as dates, time, places, spaces, period of life or the meaningful persons in question. Above all, the interviewer had to avoid reformulating in his/her own words, to avoid the trap of interpretation by reducing the subject to its own subjectivity. It should be remembered that the phenomenological interview is situated in a constructivist paradigm where, through the in-depth description of the perception of the phenomenon, the circumstances in which the symptoms (or the stroke) manifest themselves, the information gathered (or transmitted) is necessarily important and significant. This differs from positivism where the interviewer has a certain amount of specific information to collect, often using a checklist, and the interviewee tries to give the "right answers". It is therefore imperative to allow a free discourse, a dynamism of free association, where all themes are possible. We aim to avoid social desirability expressed in typical phrases such as "is this what you want me to talk about? "or "it looks like my stroke is caused by this or that". It is necessary to move away from preconceptions (prejudices) and traditional risk factor discourse to go beyond and allow the person to evoke nodes, emotional overload, events, people, relationships or meaningful dates, in short, the affective, social and symbolic environment overloaded with meaning.

Since this type of discourse's space is not a common practice, it is essential to set the table to encourage greater openness, despite the presence of possible resistance or defense mechanisms masking topics that the individual would prefer not to address. As a preamble, the interviewer reminds us that the interview remains confidential, that all topics are allowed, that we are not looking for a specific cause or answer, that the topics covered may not seem appropriate or trivial, while insisting that all associations, if disclosed, are important, that we are not looking for meaning, but rather that it is an exercise in which we express ourselves freely and in which certain emerging links may seem trivial. In this sense, the date of stroke, the details of the circumstances of its occurrence and the change in daily plans as a result of stroke have proven to be a good entry point to the horizon of signifiers perceived as individual stressors.

FOR A PHENOMENOLOGY OF STROKE

Why a phenomenology of stroke? From the point of view of knowledge transfer, this phenomenology is, first and foremost, the expression of a typical framework of a topology of the processes of symptom and disease formation. Thus, this topology could easily be applied to any form or grouping of pathologies. Let us recall, as we wrote above, that we have selected the world of the stroke especially because it occurs under the conditions of an *accident (which is not essential to the being),* fertile ground and most conducive to an interview surrounding the circumstances of its occurrence, naturally external to an intentional content, and capable of not confronting from the outset the defense mechanisms of the individual.

From a clinical point of view, the reasons for carrying out our project were twofold: firstly, from the subject's point of view, to help, as far as possible, the individual possibly affected by a stroke to go through his/her own processes of psychological elaboration and association in an attempt to deconstruct and defuse the trigger of the stroke. It should be noted that, most certainly, which we unfortunately cannot verify, several participants have already been able to defuse a future stroke simply from the space devoted to them on the subject of naïve[51] (or even pre-conscious) expression and understanding of stroke.

Then, from the perspective of the health professionals of the health care system, we simply wanted to facilitate their practical approach by introducing them to the organizational structure of stroke. In addition, on this basis, we also wanted to identify the issues of a method that could serve as a gateway to the heart of stroke development and elaboration mechanisms. By following this method, it would be simple to build a renewed interview guide that could describe the content that subjectively expresses the process of stroke formation.

According to the methodological requirements of an analytical dis-

---

51. *Naive,* that is, *representing the thing as it is.*

course, we said that our investigation is concerned with and interested in only one thing: the speech of the stroke subject. What is important here is the subject's discourse, what he/she says about stroke and its significant and symbolic environment. Why did the stroke occur under these circumstances, on this date, in this year? Only the individual can actually answer this question.

But is it real? Is it just coincidence, random? Wouldn't the person be trying to control or alleviate his/her anguish and suffering in this way by *putting* or *giving meaning* where there may not be any? Is it the song of a traveler lost in the storm? Through our space of discourse, wouldn't we give the individual the opportunity and the possibility to make connections, to pull in all directions to plug the existential gap that has opened up at the heart of the stroke?

These initial objections are recurrent, but are they well-founded? Let us say first of all, as Freud wrote in 1911[52], "that one never allows oneself to be drawn into introducing the standard of reality into morbid psychic formations; one would then run the risk of underestimating the value of associations in the formation of symptoms by invoking precisely the fact that they are not realities." Thus, the reality of what is said about stroke is not to be inferred or used as an argument here. The individual's associations, fantasies, interpretations or beliefs take precedence over everything else. As we have said over and over again, stroke is always real, like suicide, but this reality does not influence the determinations that manifest it as a phenomenon (suicide is not the reason for death).

Second, here again, as Freud[53] wrote, "It is not I who instituted the omnipotence of affects as a morbid *symptom*, it is the patient who proclaims the omnipotence in which he believes." Everything happens according to an individual's beliefs. It is no coincidence that this stroke occurred on the night of the anniversary of the murder of his spouse, it is the affective charge that this event reminds us of, an emotional charge in which the person believes to the point of putting his/her life at stake.

Third, in many cases, the participant did not know (and in many others, he/she still does not know) that it was these special circumstances that precipitated the onset of stroke. It is not essential for the ego to be aware of

---

52. "Formulation on the two principles of the course of psychic events", published in *Results, Ideas, Problems, I (1890-1920)*. Note that the citation is a free translation from French.
53. Letter to Jung dated December 19, 1901. Note that the citation is a free translation from French.

this for stroke to manifest itself; on the contrary, the defense mechanisms do everything in their power to ensure that the ego does not know anything about it.

Rather, it is on the side of the *Gegenstand,* that is, on the side of the individual's own conviction that he/she intentionally had nothing to do with the stroke, that the attempt to *make sense* of the stroke must be sought in order to come to grips with or alleviate the anguish and suffering caused by the stroke. It is on the side of reasons external to oneself that we hear the individual making connections to move away from the subjective meanings of stroke – and thus plugging the existential breach that has opened up in the heart of stroke. It is in its convictions that stroke is an extra-mental phenomenon that we hear the individual repeat, to anyone who will listen, *the stroke is not from me, it is about an order of real.*

It is therefore not through the circumstances mentioned in the interview or in the reductions made in our analysis that we can hear a misunderstanding of the subject of stroke, but rather of the extrinsic reason why the individual remains silent and patient in the face of his/her stroke. It's more in the sense that it comforts him/her.

To conclude this section, we can only corroborate Freudian theories and hear through the meaning of the manifestations of stroke a repressed node of meanings, which is expressed, secondarily, in a morbid way. The essence of this node has been described by Freud throughout his work and concerns a struggle between the satisfaction of a desire that is of the order of the unconscious and the opposition of the consciousness that refuses to recognize that it is indeed a component belonging to the ego.

In his most beautiful texts, towards the end of his work, precisely from his second topic of 1922, Freud clearly conceived that a repressed nuclear content had once been the object of a desire that had become inadmissible for the conscious ego. Thus, repressed motions concerning a death wish in relation to a same-sex parent, brother or sister, or an erotic fixation on the opposite-sex parent (or his/her representative), as well as on that brother or sister – or, even worse, as for its ravages, a homosexual fixation linked to a same-sex family member – become themes to be violently expelled from consciousness, creating an unbearable ambivalence for the balance of the individual. It is precisely the failure of this rejection outside of consciousness that will sign the pathological organization.

Here, according to Freud, it is a question of survival in the community. These motions must be repressed and supressed in order to allow the human species to exist and survive (these are the imperatives of the Law of the Unconscious concerning a double taboo prohibition and the future of the destiny of human history). In this sense, stroke is the subjective, concrete, direct and morbid consequence of this struggle.

GUIDE TO A PHENOANALYTICAL INTERVIEW ABOUT STROKE

The book concludes with a summary of the main methodological guidelines that shape phenoanalytical interviewing for health profession-als who work with individuals at risk of a second stroke. We will therefore take up the essentials expressed in the preceding sections to produce a synthesis that could eventually serve as a training guide for stakeholders interested in the phenoanalytical approach.

Let us first recall the terms of the preamble of the interviewer who initiates the phenoanalytical interview. It should be noted that the aim here is to create an unusual discourse space, which is far removed from the daily discourse and from the interview or consultation to which the person is often exposed. The aim is to introduce the space for free association on the subject of stroke and to describe how a space of discourse that goes beyond the usual framework of speaking is made available to facilitate the healthcare professional's task of entering into a phenoanalytical interview.

The preamble to the interview is intended to let the patient know that we want to take a moment to discuss and especially to hear him/her talk about the circumstances of his/her stroke. We specify that we are not looking for a cause for stroke, but simply want to describe and understand the circumstances surrounding its occurrence. We would like to take this opportunity to point out that we do not have a form to fill out, an interview grid to follow, that there are no right or wrong answers and that we want his/her version of the story. We explain, and reassure, that it may well be possible that we will address topics that, at first glance, may seem surpris-ing, stunning or seemingly unrelated directly or obviously to stroke.

To promote free association, we focus on open-ended questioning such as "Tell me…", for example, "about the occurrence of your stroke." It should also be remembered that the interviewer must be well informed about how to approach the individual's defense mechanisms so as not to confront them. In this sense, the form of a negative question such as "Nothing particularly special happened on the date of [stroke date]?" is es-pecially useful. This question allows the patient to express his/her opinion on the meaning of this date and on the particularity of this day, now and in the past. Did the stroke occur on a birthday, anniversary, celebration, important or symbolic date for the individual? The interviewer should also be alert for non-verbal cues accompanying an emotionally overinvested theme, for example, the exacerbation of tremor or repetitive nervousness movements that may be cues that the expressed content is overinvested. Excessive negation is also an indication of the presence of a theme to be repressed (remember the mathematical rule: when two negations multiply, the result is positive).

Specifically, the interviewer aims to document the specific circumstances of this stroke. To do this, he/she needs to hear the signifiers evoked by the patient as he/she tells his/her story. For example, if the patient mentions people around him/her, the interviewer will want to invite the patient to comment on the meaning of his/her relationships with these people. The same principle applies to planned activities that were cancelled due to the occurrence of the stroke. What was the meaning of these activities? Who were they to be made with? Who are these people to the patient? In short, the interviewer must be attentive to the signifiers that arise during the interview, to note the individual's symbolic environment (dates, meaningful persons, planned activities) and invite him/her to elaborate secondarily on these themes, so that the interview follows the shape of a spiral.

If we now want to define the theoretical details of our method, let's start with the example of the psychoanalytical method (which obviously cannot be used as an investigative procedure in an interview about stroke). The Freudian cure will be used here as a reference point to initiate our clinical logic. In a previously published book[54] we have tried to describe, in the simplest sense of the word, what it means to the healing experience of psychoanalysis. We said then that, if we want to specify, in three complementary and simultaneous words, the work of the cure that succeeds in disengaging the human mind from its process of symptom formation, we use the notions of *laboration, elaboration* and *perlaboration*[55].

Laboration (from labour), as the first contact with the space of analysis, inscribes in a logic of associative translation the work by which the (living) subject expresses self about a content usually expelled from the field of consciousness. It is therefore not by discussing with the consciousness – it is not by discussing with the conscious ego, by addressing our-

---

54. *Freud et l'affaire de l'inconscient.*
55. We are in line here with the logic (and beyond) of the proposed translation by Laplanche and Pontalis on the subject of *perlaboration* – the work to get through, in German *durcharbeiten* – to express the three terms of the Freudian cure: translate (*Übersetzung*), transfer (*Übertragung*) and testimony (*Überzeugung*).

selves to it – that we ask the individual to speak and that it will be possible to enter into a procedure of deconstruction of a node of the unconscious. To enter this space of discourse, the analysand, in an associative way, that is to say, outside the formal framework that prescribes communication, takes the floor to *translate* what comes to mind spontaneously, without judgement, discrimination, rationalisation or censorship. Analogically, it should be noted that a good translator directly reports the meaning of the words (signifiers) that come to him/her without interfering with the content of the translation. By association, the analysand thus speaks about his dreams, memories, impressions, desires, experiences, symptoms, fears, etc., without judging the appropriateness of the content, without separating what is real, imaginary or fantasy, without being guided by a spatial or temporal logic. The associative form of laboration thus differs from other forms of discourse in which the subject takes the floor on a daily basis; this form would be unbearable to hear on a daily basis, it has nothing to do with confidence and does not have to be narrative, argumentative, interrogative, negative, descriptive or discursive. This laboration is inscribed as a memory of the cure, in the sense that the analyst becomes the space of expression of the various representations that shape a *subject of* the unconscious.

Elaboration, as an *art of showing* in a relation of transference, is *constructed*[56] in and by the expressed content, as a double task by which analyst and analysand try to recognize the terms of resistances that inhibit the expression of this content and where the analyst, limiting self to the expressed content, shows the coherence of the links that escape consciousness, despite being explicit and recurrent in the discourse. Here we mean transfer in the sense that the content expressed is limited to the discourse of the analysand – the analytic relation being distinguished here from other spaces of discourse because we do not find the existential loop by which the subject exists by communicating with another – and where the analyst only represents the memory in which this discourse is inscribed. As with the unconscious, this memory cannot be faulty. It is a matter of know-how rather than an effort of reason.

The elaboration of the analyst's discourse interrupts in a way (*widerstand*[57], leaving in suspension, outside) the analysand's *return home to* take him/her elsewhere (precisely in the heart of the subject), where he/she

---

56. *Construction* in the Freudian sense of the 1937 text *Konstruktionen in der Analyse*.
57. *Widerstand* in the sense of resistance, but resistance to the service of analysis, against defenses of the ego.

is already, but without becoming aware of it. Let's hear *back home* in the sense of an existential loop that is omnipresent in everyday discourse and that acts as a process of censorship, an ego defense mechanism that does not allow itself to enter into the subject of the discourse or to address it.

It should be noted that the work of the cure does not in any way emphasize a communicative effect; here, there can be no question of prescription, suggestion, interpretation, intervention, that is to say, an address to the conscience to frame it, inform it, educate it, instruct it, direct it. We can say that the work of analysis leaves consciousness on the sideline[58]. Nor is the analysis addressed to the intelligence, understanding or reason of the analysand. It doesn't have to counsel him/her, refer him/her or *therapeutise* him/her. It is through this perspective that we situate *perlaboration* as a work of consciousness that recognises elaboration as its own history, that is, as a subject of the unconscious. This is how the consciousness comes to the bar (or rather to the couch) to come and *testify to the* recognition of the elaboration.

But this curative work requires a very structured, even difficult, time and space for discussion, which is not given to everyone (we speak for both the analysand and the analyst). It is here that the clinical work of the Kreuzlingen School, mainly that of Ludwig Binswanger[59] on existential analysis (*Daseinsanalysis*), can help us to design a new healing environment that partially relieves us of the requirements of Freudian cure and its transferential framework, insofar as we support it with an updated reading of the work of formal phenomenology (we naturally think of those of Husserl and Heidegger).

In brief, we can understand the clinical work of existential analysis as a process aimed first of all at putting in brackets the psychic synthesis of the patient who has led his/her existence to a systematic organization of suffering in order to substitute the process of symptom formation for a process of analysis capable of deconstructing this organization. The innovation of this process is to tone the *floating attention* of the Freudian dynamics to establish a more active interaction with the patient (which could compensate for his/her transferential lack). As we said before, as long as this clinical attitude is well defined and supported by a rigorous methodological and theoretical framework, it can only lead to satisfactory therapeutic results.

---

58. This consciousness, however, will have to be back by the time we need it for a work of perlaboration.

59. One of the most faithful and competent disciples of Freudian doctrine.

The clinical interview, which is based on a *phenoanalytical* theoretical orientation, should first be able to identify, from the individual's discourse, a network of signifiers (the vertical axis) that initiates the symptom environment, and consequently show what is actually expressed subjectively by these symptoms (the horizontal axis). Thus, the environment of stroke triggers must be identified in the person's speech at the heart of his/her pathological manifestations and not found on the basis of an interpretation proposed by an interview grid.

The first purpose of the phenoanalytical interview is therefore twofold; let us say that it is vertical and horizontal. First, the interview must identify, indicate and show the master signifiers (in Husserlian terms, *intentional objects*) that vertically trigger stroke at the particular time it occurs in an individual's life; then, it must support, inquire, investigate, always based on the patient's speech and discourse, the horizontal network of meanings (again using Husserlian terms, *intentional content*) that predisposes, organizes, develops, based on the experiences lived by the individual during his/her existence, the morbid effect that the encounter of this current signifier (intentional object) has.

When an affective predisposition, conflicting and repressed during an individual's life (horizontal predisposition), encounters a pre-signifying current situation (master signifier or vertical intentional object) and when the symbolic environment of this individual is inhabited by a phenogenesis insisting on the biogenetic inheritance of a determined pathological environment belonging to him/her (the substrate), we are then in the presence of a stroke *trigger*.

The interview, anchored by a *phenoanalytical* orientation, should thus identify a node of meanings that precedes or accompanies awareness and thematize the *pre-conscious* intentional patterns that give meaning to stroke. The important thing here is always to give the opportunity for the subject of this stroke to speak, without suggesting or framing any particular content. In this way, it is the essence of the stroke that is in question, i.e., what is most important or significant for the person's network of meanings.

Finally, it should be noted that the substrate of the stroke experience is and remains the subject's body in its reality (and in its biogenetic inheritance). The meeting of the vertical and horizontal axes merges into the real body of an individual. Stroke is of the order of a real phenomenon; it manifests itself in reality, the body of the individual suffers in its entirety, in his/her everyday life, in his/her physical and psychic reality, as well as in his/her relationship with others. What we bring to the debate is the fact that although stroke is of the order of the real, this does not alter the decisive importance of other predispositions that are of a completely different order, symbolic or environmental (psycho, phylo or phenogenetic). The fact that stroke is a real phenomenon does not make the reality the reason for it, its cause or its trigger; as a phenomenon, it cannot be its own trigger, it is influenced by various circumstances external to itself. A phenomenon cannot be its own cause or reason without admitting, *a priori*, the existence of a principle that is essentially extrinsic to it.

Let us start again from Husserl's thesis which found the phenomenological approach based on the notion of *reduction*. Starting from its principle which aims to put in brackets (*épochè*) all forms of judgments or beliefs that the existence of the object (in this case that of symptoms) is extra-mental (*Gegenstand*) – i.e., existing outside a meaningful, even intentional link. It is then that a phenomenological reduction must raise the initial expression of the object as an intentional object (*Objekt*) and hear the discourse in the sense of its intentional content. Once this reduction has been achieved, we are thus faced with a *noetic-noematic structure*[60] that leads us back to an intentional act (*Inhalt*) rather than moving away from demonstrating the true existence of the meanings of the object (i.e., the cause of stroke).

Through phenomenological reduction, the object that is supposed to be extra-mental thus manifests itself as an intentional object (*Objekt*), it becomes part of a meaningful link for consciousness, it raises its intentional content. It is here that a second reduction, an *eidetic* reduction (*eidos*, essence), is able to animate this content to raise the content of an intentional act as a pure expression of *meaning*.

The contribution of Husserlian phenomenology is fundamental to the development of our project to develop a phenoanalysis of stroke. It gives us something to think about and helps us (let us admit that this was probably not Husserl's first intention) to deconstruct the influence of biomedical discourse on the design of symptom (or even disease) formation processes.

Thus, in order to give more emphasis to the Husserlian discourse and to allow it to be in line with what we are saying, we must first put in brackets the tendency to consider the object of the discourse, here the process of stroke symptom formation, strictly as an objective phenomenon, i.e., as a biological phenomenon, real, simply accidental, predisposed only by

---

60. From *noesis* as an act turned towards the object, and *noema*, as an intentional object.

genetic heredity, outside of a meaningful universe or intentional structure. This attitude of restricting the meaning of symptoms is therefore, in Husserl's terminology, of the order of a *Gegenstand*; an extra-mental object that would stand there, in itself, as outside any form of incursion that could possibly lead us to a universe of meanings (*Bedeutungslehre*).

In a sense that bifurcates from the judgment that predisposes stroke as an accident without meaningful impact, i.e., moving away from prejudging terms such as *Gegenstände,* we must be in a position to give voice to the intentional content of stroke. We then perform a phenomenological reduction by moving the *Gegenstand* in the direction of an *Objekt, an* object of intentional content, which is affirmed in and by the patient's speech.

In line with this orientation, the heart of phenoanalysis is carried out as an interview that gives space to the intentional content of this process in the sense of an intentional act. We are then talking about the discursive effects of a second reduction, eidetic reduction, which is able to express the essence of the intentional dynamic that manifests itself through stroke.

If we indeed want to enter the subject of this process, it will be a question of *showing,* by our method, the language of the unconscious of this process (unconscious in the sense that it does not interest the conscious ego, that its contents are pushed out of consciousness), that is to say, to go in the direction of what it manifests. Only in this way will we be able to deconstruct the mechanisms of stroke symptom formation outside the time and space required by the Freudian analysis. On this basis, it will then be a matter of obtaining *confirmation*[61] from the patient that our interview is understood in the sense of an *elaborative testimony*[62] that recognizes the impact of the two reductions that express here the essential (i.e., what concerns intimately), the meaning of the stroke that is at the heart of the interview (the experience of consciousness thus confirming its conditions of possibility). Only in this way can confirmation of this elaborate testimony defuse the possible recurrence of stroke for the conscious mind.

---

61. In the sense of recognizing the construction of the elaboration of our reductions.
62. In the double sense of *Überzeugung* and *durcharbeiten*, i.e., a testimony and a perlaboration without a transferential structure.

BIBLIOGRAPHY

ADAMS, H.P. Jr., BENDIXEN, B.H., KAPPELLE, L.J., BILLER, J., LOVE, B.B., GORDON, D.L. & MARSH, E.E. 3e, (1993). Classification of subtype of acute ischemic stroke. Definitions for use in a multicenter clinical trial. TOAST. Trial of Org 10172 in Acute Stroke Treatment. *Stroke, 24,* 35-41.

BARKER, W.H. & MULLOOLY, J.P. (1997). Stroke in a defined elderly population, 1967-1985. A less lethal and disabling but no less common disease. *Stroke, 28,* 284-290.

BINSWANGER, L. (1971). *Introduction à l'analyse existentielle.* Les Éditions de Minuit.

BINSWANGER, L. (1970) *Analyse existentielle et psychanalyse freudienne.* Éditions Gallimard.

DESCARTES, R. (1960). *Discours de la Méthode.* Éditions Garnier Frères.

DESROSIERS, J., NOREAU, L., ROCHETTE, A., BRAVO, G. & BOUTIN, C. (2002). Predictors of handicap situations following post-stroke rehabilitation. *Disabil Rehabil, 24,* 774-785.

ENGSTROM, G., KHAN, F.A., ZIA, E., JERNTORP, I, PESSAH-RASMUSSEN, H., NORRVING, B. & JANZON, L. (2004). Marital dissolution is followed by an increased incidence of stroke. *Cerebrovasc Dis, 18,* 318-324.

FEIGIN, V.L., LAWES, C.M., BENNETT, D.A. & ANDERSON, C.S. (2003). Stroke epidemiology: a review of population-based studies of incidence, prevalence, and case-fatality in the late 20th century. *Lancet Neurol, 2,* 43-53.

Fondation des maladies du coeur du Canada. [on-line] www.fmcoeur.qc.ca/ [as accessed 9 June 2015].

FOUGEYROLLAS, P. (1995). Documenting environmental factors for preventing the handicap creation process: Quebec contributions relating to ICIDH and social participation of people with functional differences. *Disabil Rehabil, 17,* 145-53.

FREUD, A. (1972). *Le Moi et les mécanismes de défense.* PUF.

FREUD, S. (1984). *Résultats, idées, problèmes, I (1890-1920).* PUF.

- (1981). *Névrose, psychose et perversion*. PUF.

- (1980). *L'interprétation des rêves*. PUF.

- (1977). *La technique psychanalytique*. PUF.

- (1979). *Cinq psychanalyses*. PUF.

- (1980). *Totem et tabou*. Petite Bibliothèque Payot, no 77.

- (1940). *Métapsychologie*. Éditions Gallimard.

- (1980). *Essai de psychanalyse*. Petite Bibliothèque Payot, no 44.

- (1981). *Inhibition, symptôme et angoisse*. PUF.

FREUD, S. & BULLIT, W.C. (1967). *Le président Wilson*. Éditions Albin Michel.

FREUD, S. & C.G. JUNG, C.G. (1975). *Correspondance, I (1906-1909)*. Gallimard, coll. NRF.

GAULIN, P. (1988). D'un problème homosexuel non résolu à la réussite là où le paranoïaque échoue. *Revue clinique méditerranéenne*, 17-18, 227-243.

GAULIN, P., DUBÉ, M., HAMEL, S. & LEFRANÇOIS, R. (2002). Répondants défensifs et désirabilité sociale des plus âgés: une certaine conséquence associée à l'organisation de la société techno-médicale. *Revue québécoise de psychologie*, 23, (2), 73-85.

GAULIN, P. (2003). *Le Culte technomédical : approche psychanalytique. Le prix à payer pour que le verbe se fasse chair*. Les éditions Triptyque.

GAULIN, P. (2006). *Traiter, cent ans après la psychanalyse de Freud, dans une société technomédicale*. Les éditions Triptyque.

GAULIN, P. (2010a). *Freud et l'affaire de l'inconscient. L'espace subjectif dans la société technomédicale et virtuelle (psychanalyse du virtuel)*. Les éditions Triptyque.

GAULIN, P. (2010b). *Freud et la philosophie*, texte intégral d'une conférence, dans *La mort, Séminaire 1985-1988* de François Péraldi. Éditons Liber (Voix psychanalytiques).

GORDON, D.L., BENDIXEN, B.H., ADAMS, H.P.Jr., CLARKE, W., KAPPELLE, L.J. & WOOLSON, R.F. (1993). Interphysician agreement in the diagnosis of subtypes of acute ischemic stroke : implications for clinical trials. The TOAST Investigators. *Neurology,* 43, 1021-1027.

HAAPANIEMI, H., HILLBOM, M. & JUVELA, S. (1996). Weekend and holiday increase in the onset of ischemic stroke in young women. *Stroke,* 27, 1023-1027.

HARDIE, K., HANKEY, G.J., JAMROZIK, K., BROADHURST, R.J. & ANDERSON, C. (2004). Ten-year risk of first recurrent stroke and disability after first-ever stroke in the Perth Community Stroke Study. *Stroke,* 35, 731-735.

HEGEL, G.W.F. (2006). *Phénoménologie de l'esprit.* Vrin.

HEGEL, G.W.F. (1970). *Encyclopédie des sciences philosophiques, I. La science de la logique.* Vrin.

HEIDEGGER, M. (1976). *Acheminement vers la parole.* Éditions Gallimard.

HEIDEGGER, M. (1958). *Essais et conférences.* Gallimard, coll. NRF.

HUSSERL, E. (1950). *Idées directrices pour une phénoménologie.* Éditions Gallimard.

HUSSERL, E. (1953). *Méditations cartésiennes. Introduction à la phénoménologie.* Vrin.

HUSSERL, E. (2009). *Recherches logiques, 1, 2-1, 2-2, 3.* PUF.

KANT, E. (1984). *Critique de la raison pure.* Quadrigue et PUF.

KOTON, S., TANNE, D., BORNSTEIN, N.M. & GREEN, M.S. (2004). Triggering risk factors for ischemic stroke: a case-crossover study. *Neurology,* 63, 2006-2010.

LACAN, J. (1966). *Écrits.* Éditions du Seuil.

OMS. (2001). *Classification internationale du fonctionnement, du handicap et de la santé.* [on-line] http ://apps.who.int/classifications/icfbrowser/.

PATTON, M. (2002). *Qualitative Research & Evaluation Methods.* Sage Publications.

PLATON. (1968) *La République.* Éditions Gonthier.

POUPART, J., DESLAURIERS, J.-P., GROULX, L.-H., LAPERRIÈRE, A., MAYER, R. & PIRES, A. (1997). *La recherche qualitative : enjeux épistémologiques et méthodologiques.* G.M. éditeur.

Réseau international sur le processus de production du handicap. [on-line] http:// www.ripph.qc.ca/.

ROCHETTE, A., DESROSIERS, J., BRAVO, G., ST-CYR-TRIBBLE, D. & BOURGET, A. (2007a). Changes in participation after a mild stroke: quantitative and qualitative perspectives. *Top Stroke Rehabil,* 14, 59-68.

ROCHETTE, A., DESROSIERS, J., BRAVO, G., TRIBBLE, D.S. & BOURGET, A. (2007b). Changes in participation level after spouse's first stroke and relationship to burden and depressive symptoms. *Cerebrovasc Dis,* 24, 255-60.

ROCHETTE, A., DESROSIERS, J. & NOREAU, L. (2001). Association between personal and environmental factors and the occurrence of handicap situations following a stroke. *Disabil Rehabil,* 23, 559-569.

ROCHETTE, A., GAULIN, P. & TELLIER, M. (2009). Could stroke trigger be prevented by healthy family relationships? *Int J Rehabil Res,* 32, 173-177.

ROCHETTE, A., KORNER-BITENSKY, N., BISHOP, D., TEASELL, R., WHITE, C.L., BRAVO, G., COTE, R., GREEN, T., LEBRUN, L.H., LANTHIER, S., KAPRAL, M. & BAYLEY, M. (2013). The YOU CALL-WE CALL Randomized Clinical Trial: Impact of a Multimodal Support Intervention After a Mild Stroke. *Circ Cardiovasc Qual Outcomes,* 6, 674-679.

SAPOSNIK, G., BAIBERGENOVA, A., DANG, J. & V. HACHINSKI, V. (2006). Does a birthday predispose to vascular events? *Neurology,* 67, 300-304.

STALNIKOWICZ, R. & TSAFRIR, A. (2002). Acute psychosocial stress and cardiovascular events. *Am J Emerg Med,* 20, 488-491.

STRAUS, S.E., MAJUMDAR, S.R. & MCALISTER, F.A. (2002). New evidence for stroke prevention : clinical applications. *Jama,* 288, 1396-1398.

TANNE, D., GOLDBOURT, U. & MEDALIE, J.H. (2004). Perceived family difficulties and prediction of 23-year stroke mortality among middle-aged men. *Cerebrovasc Dis,* 18, 277-282.

VINCENT, C., DEAUDELIN, I., ROBICHAUD, L., ROUSSEAU, J., VISCOGLIOSI, C., TALBOT, L.R. & DESROSIERS, J. (2007). Rehabilitation needs for older adults with stroke living at home : perceptions of four populations. *BMC Geriatr,* 7, 20.

ACKNOWLEDGEMENTS

We sincerely thank the professionals, members of the research team, all affiliated with the Centre hospitalier universitaire de Montréal (CHUM Notre-Dame): Dr. Laury Chamelian (neuro-psychiatrist), Lucie Hébert (Ph.D. occupational therapist), Marlène Lapierre (research nurse) and Dr. Yan Deschaintre (neurologist). Finally, we would also like to thank the study participants who spoke about the circumstances surrounding the occurrence of their stroke.

www.ingramcontent.com/pod-product-compliance
Lightning Source LLC
Chambersburg PA
CBHW070928270326
41927CB00011B/2771